T0281728

WELCOMING LGBT RESIDENTS

Welcoming LGBT Residents is the first comprehensive guide to working with LGBT older adults in senior living settings.

The LGBT older adult population represents one of the fastest-growing subpopulations within our aging society. Despite the increasing demand for LGBT-affirming services there is an absence of training books for care providers. This dual-purpose text is appropriate for training and as a guide to answer questions that may come up during daily tasks. It is based on the most recent research and includes stories and testimonials from LGBT older adults and providers in the field. Chapters include

- LGBT-inclusive intake and conversations;
- Gender identity and expression;
- Memory care and LGBT people;
- Navigating family dynamics;
- Addressing conflict between residents;
- Staff opinions, beliefs, and training.

This timely book will be of interest to professional care providers, from long-term care nurses and assisted living administrators to staff in retirement communities, as well as students in gerontology, health care administration, and social work courses.

Tim R. Johnston is the Senior Director of National Projects for SAGE, the country's largest and oldest organization dedicated to improving the lives of LGBT older people.

"Tim Johnston's book is a timely, grounded, and most importantly useful guide for how to make our services more open to LGBT seniors. It can serve as a reference text for leadership staff and also an accessible educational tool for students and staff. I would encourage anyone working with older adults, not only those working in senior living, to take a look and see what they can learn."

—Paula Basta, Director of the Illinois Department of Aging
and Former Chair of the LGBT Aging Issues
Network of the American Society on Aging

"For far too long, LGBT older people have encountered bias, stigma, and discrimination across the senior living environment. In response to this profound problem, Tim Johnston has written a comprehensive and accessible resource for the entire eldercare workforce—one that acknowledges that many LGBT older people live at the intersection of multiple identities, and they, as much as anyone, deserve to have a place they can call 'home.'"

—Robert Espinoza, Vice President of Policy, PHI

"Combining current research, best practices, and his own experiences training providers across the country, Dr Johnston has created a road map for providers of services and supports to create safe and affirming environments where LGBTQ older adults can thrive. This comprehensive text is a valuable guide and resource for any provider looking to make their organization a place where older adults, their families and staff can be who they are, regardless of their sexual orientation or gender identity."

—Kevin Bradley, Associate Director of Online Learning, LeadingAge

"With an extensive background in advocacy and training, the author has significant experience and working knowledge of the needs of older LGBT adults. The history of LGBT people includes discrimination, criminality, being considered deviant or mentally ill and subjected to inappropriate medical 'therapies'. This, coupled with the dearth of research into the needs of older LGBT adults, makes this publication most welcome. Raising awareness of the uniqueness of each person and alerting care providers to the fact that LGBT people are not a homogenous group can only be a positive contributor to the provision of 'safer and more inclusive spaces'."

—Patricia MacGabhann BNS (Hons) HDip Gerontology MSc Science
MHSc Specialist Nursing (National University of Ireland, Galway),
Clinical and Operational Director, Nightingale Nursing Home

"This book presents significant insights into creating inclusive environments for older LGBT people. It will also enable professionals to respond appropriately to challenging situations in residential care homes."

—Dr Ralf Lottmann, Marie Skłodowska-Curie Fellow at the
University of Surrey, UK (Research Project: 'Ageing & Diversity:
LGBT* Housing and Long-term Care')

WELCOMING LGBT RESIDENTS

A Practical Guide for Senior Living Staff

TIM R. JOHNSTON

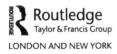

Routledge
Taylor & Francis Group

LONDON AND NEW YORK

First published 2020
by Routledge
2 Park Square, Milton Park, Abingdon, Oxon OX14 4RN

and by Routledge
52 Vanderbilt Avenue, New York, NY 10017

Routledge is an imprint of the Taylor & Francis Group, an informa business

© 2020 Tim R. Johnston

British Library Cataloguing-in-Publication Data
A catalogue record for this book is available from the British Library

Library of Congress Cataloging-in-Publication Data
A catalog record has been requested for this book

ISBN: 978-0-367-02732-2 (hbk)
ISBN: 978-0-367-02734-6 (pbk)
ISBN: 978-0-429-39813-1 (ebk)

Typeset in Sabon
by Apex CoVantage, LLC

CONTENTS

DEDICATION AND ACKNOWLEDGMENTS

This book is dedicated to the LGBT older adults, activists, and allies working every day to make sure we can all live with dignity as we age. I want to give special thanks to my colleagues at SAGE and the network of trainers who are the heart and soul of the SAGECare training program.

Thank you to the many colleagues, reviewers, friends, and contributors who added their perspectives and voices to this book, as well as Chris Moyer for creating the cover image. Special thanks to the following people for providing feedback on specific chapters: Mark Brennan-Ing, Terri Clark, Heather Finkelston, Maureen Garvey, Nancy Giunta, Rene Hickman, Britta Larson, Celia Laskey, Jonathan Malamy, Cheryl Martin, Kelly Ording, Shannon Ruedlinger, Erica Steelman, and Aaron Tax. I would also like to thank the anonymous reviewers who provided thoughtful feedback, as well as those who have written endorsements for the book.

Finally—thank you to my partner, Daniel Susser. I don't know if our journey will lead us to a senior living community, but I guarantee you if it does, it'll be a community that has drag queen bingo.

FOREWORD

In 2014, with support from executive leadership, I initiated Abramson Senior Care's efforts to become more welcoming, affirming and competent in providing care and services to LGBT+ older adults. I didn't realize then, and now reflect with pride and gratitude, that while forging an uncharted path for our organization, I would join a growing group of dedicated individuals working to make medical and long-term care service providers aware of, sensitive to, and resourceful in providing optimal care for all, including LGBT+ older adults.

One of the first things I did was create the LGBT+ Task Force, which continues to this day, with staff from different departments and positions throughout our organization and a resident representative. We had an idea of where we wanted to end up, but how would an organization with a 150-year history go from point A to point B?

I searched for resources and models and quickly confirmed that there was a dearth of research on older LGBT+ adults. Furthermore, there was very little information to guide long-term care providers.

This did not deter me. While working as a chaplain and a member of our interdisciplinary care team, I began to talk openly about the existence of LGBT+ people and to normalize discussing sexuality, sexual orientation, and gender identity. I developed a conceptual framework for understanding person-centered care that incorporates an awareness of and sensitivity to sexual orientation and gender identity as core components of a person. I started giving presentations on person-centered care for LGBT+ older adults to members of the Abramson Senior Care community and beyond in other academic and professional settings. It's been exciting to see these ideas catch on and interest in doing this work spread.

At the core of true person-centered care is the understanding that each person is a unique, multidimensional, complex being, as well as the recognition of our shared humanity. We have the honor and privilege to be part of caring professions. People, often in their most vulnerable states, are in our care, and as such it behooves us to do all we can to provide sensitive, compassionate, competent services and care. But how do we do this as individuals and organizations?

Shortly after forming our LGBT+ Task Force, I met Dr. Tim Johnston and discussed this question. It has been my pleasure to know and work with him over the past five years on the shared goal of improving services and care for LGBT+ older adults. From our initial conversation, I experienced his thoughtfulness and keen intellect, both of which are reflected throughout this book. His insight and support have been invaluable.

Dr. Johnston, in writing this book, has helped fill the void that has existed until now. Unlike when I began our LGBT+ Initiatives, you can find in this publication a wealth of information and resources on providing care and services to LGBT+ older adults in long-term care settings. Because Dr. Johnston appreciates each organization is unique and dynamic, he discusses options and opportunities for creating change. He provides resources for you to have at hand as you think through what steps you and your organization might take.

Another major contribution of this book stems from Dr. Johnston's awareness of and sensitivity to the ways in which differences exist in terms of the experiences of sub-groups within the larger LGBT+ group. Dr. Johnston's commitment in allowing previously silent voices to have a platform is significant. For instance, he has devoted Chapter 9 to bisexuality and aging to bring awareness and understanding to a historically overlooked and misunderstood sexual orientation and population. On p. 67, he explains that there is long-standing prejudice against bisexuality and bisexuals, both among LGBT+ people and in mainstream society.

Dr. Johnston has gathered helpful insights and reflections from older LGBT+ adults as well as from practitioners who work with older adults. For instance, Dr. Erin Partridge's discussion (p. 30) of how she handles personal questions is an eloquent and poignant reminder that the decision to disclose one's sexual orientation and/or gender identity is a personal decision for both staff and residents, and people may choose, for different reasons, what and what not to disclose. The key is for people to feel comfortable in sharing as much as they want of who they are with their care team so as to be as healthy and fulfilled as possible.

You will be surprised by how many people benefit both directly and indirectly from doing the work to become more sensitive and culturally-aware to the needs of LGBT+ individuals and families. For while LGBT+ people are a minority, many heterosexual and/or cisgender individuals have people in their lives who are LGBT+. Since starting our LGBT+ Task Force, I have had staff from throughout the organization, family members, residents, and volunteers share stories of their personal connection to this work as someone who either is LGBT+ or has a personal connection to someone who is LGBT+. The sense of relief and gratitude they have expressed in being able to talk to me about their thoughts, feelings, and experiences cannot be overstated. There has been such stigma, shame, and fear surrounding LGBT+ people and families that many have struggled alone.

Often, you will not be aware of the ways your work positively impacts others, and then sometimes you will discover this, perhaps when you least expect it. On p. 16, I share one such experience that came about through our Pride Month commemorations.

As someone engaged in this work, I encourage you to be compassionate with yourself and those you work with. It is interdisciplinary in nature and rooted in collaborative efforts. And while it can be challenging, it is important and essential to providing optimal care. I wholeheartedly believe that in doing this work, you will grow personally and provide better care. Institutionally, your organization will benefit by making people feel welcomed, valued, and affirmed. For example, talented staff members have told me that they chose to work for Abramson Senior Care over other comparable opportunities because of our LGBT+ Task Force.

I now understand that we never fully arrive at the so-called point B. Rather, this work is ongoing as we strive for an aspirational destination. Dr. Tim Johnston's book can be your companion on this journey. It can offer insights, suggestions, and encouragement as you and your organization thoughtfully and responsibly make changes that will benefit your organization and the people you serve. Whatever your role is you can find useful information in this insightful book. *You* can make a difference. Organizational and personal change in this area are possible, and taking the time to read and engage with this book is an excellent first step! Wishing you all the best on your journey.

Rabbi Erica Steelman, MAHL, MPP
Director of LGBT+ Initiatives, Staff Chaplain
Abramson Center for Jewish Life

INTRODUCTION

How to read this book

Let me begin by saying that I am so excited you are interested in learning more about LGBT inclusion and LGBT older adults!

I am a full-time advocate for LGBT older adults, and in this role I have trained providers across the United States. I have walked into classrooms where people are excited about what I have to say, and I've trained groups who meet me with aggressive and combative comments. I have worked in high-end retirement communities with yoga studios and fine dining, and I've spent lots of time in memory care, assisted living, and skilled nursing facilities. Over the years I have trained, coached, and advised thousands of people, and been asked every question you can imagine.

All of that is to say, I have a lot of experience with what LGBT inclusion looks like in the field, and I'm excited to share what I've learned, and many other resources, to help you and your staff do the work of creating safer spaces for LGBT residents.

I am writing this book with a commitment to taking an intersectional approach to human identities. First coined by Kimberlé Crenshaw (1989), "intersectionality" refers to the fact that each person has many different identities that intersect within us. This is an important commitment if we are to avoid treating LGBT older adults as a homogeneous or monolithic group. I think this quote does a nice job of demonstrating the importance of intersectionality:

> Discrimination occurs among most LGBT older adults; however, vast intragroup differences exist and are related to disability, age, gender status, race, income, the quality of aging, and identity development. An LGBT older adult, who is transgender, single, working class, a person of color, and resides with friends in an apartment, lives in a society where his or her gender, sexuality, and marital status are inconsistent with cultural values such as patriarchy, heterosexual marriage, home ownership, economic success, and reproduction. Conversely, the middle-class gay male, who is married to and living with his husband, has children, and owns a home, occupies identity statuses that are culturally privileged and valued.
>
> (Robinson-Wood and Weber 2016, 66)

Taking an intersectional approach means being aware of how these differences impact people's experiences, and how they should guide providers as they create safer and more inclusive spaces.

Each chapter centers on a particular topic or aspect of senior living. Within the chapter I point out how the topic relates to LGBT people and how the discussion is impacted by other identities, such as race, ethnicity, religion, ability, immigration status, geographic location, and economic status. At times I speak of the LGBT community as a general category, and at times I will be more specific and discuss people's experiences according to gender identity or sexual orientation. When I do discuss specific identities, it is often to point out disparities in health, income, or other structural challenges to aging well.

Another important concept is that of minority stress. Developed by Ilan H. Meyer (2003), minority stress explains how living in a social environment full of stigma, stress, discrimination, and violence can lead to poor health outcomes for people in minority groups. This is important because I want to be clear that there isn't anything about being LGBT that predisposes or causes a person to be less healthy or face challenges. Instead, the disparities we will discuss are often the result of living in a world that was, and continues to be, hostile to LGBT people.

The information and recommendations in this book are based in current academic research, best practices suggested by practitioners and advocates, and my own experience training providers across the country. I have also solicited real-life examples, suggestions, testimonials, stories, and other information from a national survey of providers, LGBT older adults, family members, and advocates. Many of the contributors wanted to be named in the text; others did not, and in some circumstances I have changed names or details to protect their privacy. I hope that including on-the-ground voices of those living and working in senior living communities helps round out the book and will resonate with your work.

The topics I discuss, my resources, the questions I address, and what I emphasize are all drawn from my experience and necessarily reflect my expertise but also my biases, omissions and assumptions. That is to say, my own perspective and experiences in the field have shaped what you will find in this book, and it is not meant to be the definitive book on LGBT inclusion. Rather, what you will find is a collection of topics, ideas, and suggestions that continues the already-vibrant conversation about LGBT inclusion in senior living spaces.

EMPOWERING RESIDENT CHOICE

Our goal as providers is to maximize each resident's ability to make their own choices and have as much autonomy as possible. They are the experts on how they want to live life, not us. This also applies to whether or not someone wants to come out and openly identify as LGBT. The suggestions in this book are intended to remove any barriers that might keep a resident from coming out, but we must never pressure or force anyone to come out if they do not want to do so. It might be the case that you and your staff make all of the changes I suggest and nobody comes out, at least not right away. Do not let that discourage you. Even if a resident makes the decision to remain private about who they are, I am certain they will see the work you are doing and appreciate it. They might not decide to come out, but they will likely feel more secure, more comfortable, and more appreciated.

HOW TO READ THIS BOOK

The chapters in this book are written to be read in order, but each stands alone and is designed to address thematic areas and questions and provide information, suggestions, and additional resources. Many of the key concepts and terminology are introduced in Chapters 1 and 2, so I recommend starting with those chapters before moving on to others. This book is geared toward staff working in any kind of senior living community, from retirement communities and independent living to assisted living, memory care, skilled nursing, and short-term rehabilitation. I am focused on this aspect of aging network services because senior living staff are working in and helping to create spaces that are residents' homes. This is a unique honor and responsibility, and creating inclusive and safe homes for LGBT older adults is foundational to their wellbeing.

While senior living staff are the primary audience for this book it will be useful to anyone working with older adults, as well as for LGBT older adults and their advocates. Many of these suggestions for LGBT inclusion in senior living can be translated into other services. For example, LGBT-inclusive intake interviewing is a skill that can be used across many services.

Likewise, LGBT marketing and outreach techniques, or ways to incorporate LGBT inclusion into strategic planning, are not specific to senior living and can be used across many different businesses. LGBT older adults and advocates can use the suggestions in this book as a checklist of things to look for during tours, as well as questions to ask when shopping around for housing or other providers. For example, they can ask if the staff has been trained on LGBT cultural competency, if the nondiscrimination policy is LGBT-inclusive, and whether the community has any kind of LGBT-themed or inclusive programming.

Chapters 1 through 4 offer some suggestions for marketing, policies, programming, and move-in. The suggestions in these chapters will help you to attract new LGBT residents and to create services and spaces that send welcoming messages to your current residents. Chapters 5 to 7 look at various spaces where conflict may emerge, including how to train staff, address bullying, and navigate family dynamics. Chapters 8 through 12 turn to some psychosocial and health considerations for residents, including sexuality, gender identity, dementia, and HIV/AIDS. I decided to create standalone chapters for bisexuality and older people living with HIV because both are underdiscussed topics in LGBT aging activism and I wanted to draw special attention to these members of our community. The final chapters look at legal protections, policy, and strategic planning.

Each chapter begins with learning objectives and is divided into sub-headings for easy navigation. At the end of each chapter I summarize suggestions and key take-aways and point to resources for further reading and research. I hope that you find this book helpful, and once again I thank you for your interest in creating spaces where we can all be our full selves.

REFERENCES

Crenshaw, Kimberlé. 1989. "Demarginalizing the Intersection of Race and Sex: A Black Feminist Critique of Antidiscrimination Doctrine, Feminist Theory and Antiracist Politics." *University of Chicago Legal Forum* 1989 (1): 139–67.

Meyer, Ilan H. 2003. "Prejudice, Social Stress, and Mental Health in Lesbian, Gay, and Bisexual Populations: Conceptual Issues and Research Evidence." *Psychological Bulletin* 129 (5): 674–97. https://doi.org/10.1037/0033-2909.129.5.674.

Robinson-Wood, Tracy, and Amanda Weber. 2016. "Deconstructing Multiple Oppressions Among LGBT Older Adults." In *Handbook of LGBT Elders*, edited by Debra A. Harley and Pamela B. Teaster, 65–81. Cham: Springer International Publishing. https://doi.org/10.1007/978-3-319-03623-6.

GETTING TO KNOW LGBT OLDER ADULTS

SUMMARY

LGBT older adults are a growing part of senior living communities, but they are often invisible because they may hide their identities and relationships and because many staff assume all residents are heterosexual and cisgender. People working in any kind of senior living environment, from retirement communities to skilled nursing and memory care, have the opportunity to create a space for LGBT older adults to be open about who they are. This chapter presents some statistics and information about LGBT older adults and also orients the reader to appropriate and inappropriate terminology and the major events of LGBT history in the United States.

OBJECTIVES

- Learn key facts and figures related to the size of the LGBT older adult population, where they live, and their unique needs and concerns.
- Get comfortable with affirming terminology and learn some words to avoid when working with LGBT older adults.
- Understand how the history of oppression and discrimination experienced by the LGBT community may make LGBT older adults less willing to come out in your community or to staff.
- Consider how being LGBT intersects with other identities, such as race, ethnicity, religion, age, and country of origin.

WE WORK IN THEIR HOME

Several years ago I was training staff at a skilled nursing facility, and when I posed the question, "Why is it important that we provide sensitive care?" one of the staff members responded, "Because to me this place may just be where I work—but for our residents this is their home."

I have heard that sentiment many times over the years, and it is particularly important when we consider that often the only place where LGBT people feel completely comfortable and relaxed is at home. They may not be openly LGBT at work or with their families or friends, and may feel stressed when interacting with strangers or new people. If this is the case, it is often at home where LGBT people can let down their guard and finally relax.

This is one of the reasons that many LGBT people are petrified at the thought of moving into any kind of senior living environment. Privacy can be hard to find in many communities, and giving up that safe space may mean giving up the one place they can be themselves. For reasons I discuss in the following sections, many LGBT older adults also fear unequal or discriminatory treatment, in addition to worrying if they will have any place left where they can be themselves.

Staff can make all the difference. If residents know that they are accepted and supported by staff, they can flourish. They will maintain important relationships, develop new friendships or loves, and generally be themselves in their new community. If we get it right, working in an LGBT resident's home can be a gift—the opportunity to help them create their ideal home.

HOW MANY LGBT SENIORS ARE THERE, AND WHERE DO THEY LIVE?

This important question is difficult to answer. Very few survey or census tools ask questions about sexual orientation and gender identity. Some older adults are afraid to disclose that information, or they may engage in same-sex sexual activity but not identify as LGBT. That said, by best estimates there are 2.7 million people over the age of 50 who identify as LGBT, 1.1 million of whom are over the age of 65 (Fredriksen-Goldsen 2016, 6). To put that in perspective, the population of Chicago is 2.7 million people (U.S. Census Bureau n.d.). By 2060, the number of LGBT older adults is expected to reach 5 million, and the estimate could more than double if you include people who are in same-sex relationships but do not self-identify as LGBT or who report same sex attractions (Fredriksen-Goldsen and Kim 2017, S1). For example, around 19 million Americans (or 8.2 percent) reported having engaged in same-sex sexual behavior, and 25.6 million (or 11 percent) report some same-sex attraction (Robinson-Wood and Weber 2016). This is a large segment of the growing senior population, and LGBT people are looking for communities where they can be open.

There is an incorrect stereotype that LGBT people all move to big cities. In fact, LGBT people live in every community across the country. A report by the Williams Institute at UCLA found that the percentages of LGB people in California living in urban versus rural settings more or less matched the percentages of non-LGB people in those places (the authors did not have enough data to include transgender older adults in this analysis; Meyer, Choi, and Kittle 2018). While it is true that there are often large LGBT communities in major cities, LGBT people are everywhere. Whether your community is in San Francisco or in the heart of Appalachia it almost certainly has or has had LGBT residents.

People who do not have LGBT friends or family members learn about our communities from the media, and many of the most famous LGBT older people, like Ellen DeGeneres and Caitlyn Jenner, are white. LGBT people are a part of all other communities, which means that the LGBT older adult population is just as diverse as the United States as a whole. The number of racially and ethnically diverse LGBT characters in popular media is increasing: in the 2018–19 season 50 percent of LGBT characters on broadcast television and 46 percent on cable were people of color, a 14- and 11-point increase respectively (GLAAD 2018). This marks a significant increase from previous years and more accurately reflects the diversity of the LGBT community, but the historical absence of LGBT people of color in the media means that many people have little or no idea of the diversity within the LGBT community. Researchers estimate that approximately 20 percent of the total population of LGBT older adults are people of color (Kim et al. 2016, 49). Many of these elders have had to deal with stigmas related to their LGBT identity in addition to racism and racial discrimination. This results in some unique challenges. For example, older African-American and Hispanic LGBT adults report lower household incomes, education levels, and social supports (Kim, Jen, and Fredriksen-Goldsen 2017). Not all immigrants are people of color but many are, and it is estimated that there are 140,800 documented LGBT immigrants over the age of 55 in the United States, and 10,000 LGBT people over 55 who are undocumented (Gates 2013). These older adults face stressors related to being LGBT as well as anti-immigrant sentiment and policies. Beyond race and nationality, LGBT people are a part of every religious community, socioeconomic class, and other aspects of our intersectional identities.

Over the past 30 years, advocates for LGBT older adults have been primarily concerned with members of the Greatest Generation (people born roughly between 1914 and 1924), and the Silent Generation (1924–1945). Now providers are shifting to work with Baby Boomers (1945–1964). Baby Boomers are seen as more independent and comfortable asking for what they want. LGBT Baby Boomers may have come out earlier in life and be strong advocates for their own interests. These are broad generalizations, but over the next 15 years we are likely to see interesting shifts in what both LGBT and non-LGBT residents expect from senior living communities and providers.

HETEROSEXISM, CISSEXISM, AND LGBT OLDER ADULT INVISIBILITY

Given that there are so many LGBT older adults in all of our communities, I'm always surprised when I tell people that I work with LGBT older adults and their response is, "Wow, I've never thought about LGBT people getting older!"

This reaction says something important about LGBT older adults: they are often invisible. One reason older adults may be invisible is that they are hiding their identities. When entering a new space many LGBT older adults hide their identity or go back in the closet because they are concerned about being treated poorly. One study found that 82 percent of respondents reported being victimized at least once in their life, and 64 percent experienced victimization at least three times. This victimization includes verbal and physical assault, being hassled by police, or having their property damaged. Moreover, transgender older adults were victimized at higher rates than non-transgender older adults (Fredriksen-Goldsen 2011). One survey of LGBT and non-LGBT older adults living in long-term care communities found that 89 percent predicted that staff would discriminate against an LGBT resident, and 77 percent said they thought other residents would isolate an LGBT resident (Justice in Aging et al. 2015, 9). Another survey found that 40 percent of LGBT older adults report that their networks are getting smaller, compared to only 27 percent of non-LGBT older adults (Espinoza 2014), and studies have found that LGBT older adults are more isolated and report higher rates of loneliness than their peers (Choi and Meyer 2016). For more on the social networks of LGBT older adults see Kim et al. 2017.

There is ageism within the LGBT community as well, and when LGBT organizations or community centers focus on youth they may also inadvertently contribute to making older LGBT people feel invisible. If you do not think that you have any LGBT residents living in your community, it may be that LGBT residents are simply afraid to discuss their identity. For an overview of the academic literature on LGBT older adults in long-term care, staff opinions and training, and the impact of homophobia and heterosexism on the long-term care environment see Schwinn and Dinkel 2015.

BOX 1.1 "WHAT WOULD YOU LOOK FOR IN A RETIREMENT COMMUNITY?"

I asked Ellen Wong, who identifies as a lesbian Generation Xer, what she would look for in a potential retirement community:

> First, I'd want to know if I can afford it. Second, how diverse are the residents? And third, what services—like a gym, entertainment, or clubs—does the community provide? In order to determine the diversity and therefore tolerance level, I would look for the rainbow flag, if there is a PFLAG chapter on campus, what kind of groups or clubs were listed on the website or materials. It would be important for me to see the words 'Welcoming,' and 'Diversity' used in their publicity materials.

Another reason that LGBT older adults are invisible is that we live in a heterosexist and cissexist society, and people tend to assume that older people are not LGBT. By "heterosexist" I mean the idea that everyone is or should be heterosexual. Cissexism is the belief that everyone is or should be cisgender (i.e. not transgender—for more on the word "cisgender" see the next section and Chapter 10). When a receptionist asks an older woman if she has a husband, that is a heterosexist assumption that she is heterosexual. When a programming volunteer assumes which bathroom a person will use based on their appearance, that may reflect cissexism, because they assume that certain aspects of our appearance mean a person identifies with a particular gender identity. I do not introduce these words to place blame or admonish anyone but to help us reflect on the fact that we make many assumptions, and much of how we organize and run senior living organizations may reinforce rather than question those assumptions. If a staff person makes an assumption that a resident is heterosexual and/or cisgender, that resident is now in the position of needing to correct the staff, which the resident may decide is too risky. Many of the suggestions in this book are intended to help make us all more sensitive to these assumptions and give residents the space to tell us who they are and how they identify.

The other response I hear in my trainings is, "I treat everyone the same; what does it matter if someone is LGBT?" While it is a good goal to treat everyone the same, LGBT older adults have many specific concerns about their safety, disparities in health and income, and unique social and support networks. It is helpful to draw a distinction between equality and equity. Treating everyone equally means treating everyone in exactly the same manner, regardless of their individual needs or abilities. Treating people equitably means providing them with the individualized supports they need in order to thrive.

For example, in Figure 1.1 giving everyone the same bicycle is technically treating them equally, but the bicycle does not match their specific needs. Equity is giving everyone a bicycle that they can use, allowing them all to ride.

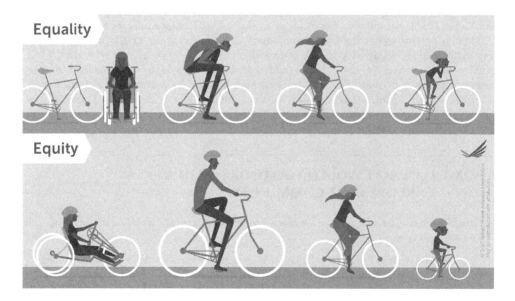

Figure 1.1 Equality versus equity

© 2017 Robert Wood Johnson Foundation

Knowing that a person is LGBT can tell you important information about their personal experiences, history, relationships, and how they want to live their life. The goal of this book is not to convince anyone that LGBT older adults deserve some kind of special treatment but rather to give staff the skills and information they need to provide LGBT residents with person-directed care, tailored to each resident as an individual.

USING LGBT-AFFIRMING TERMINOLOGY

Many people want to treat LGBT people with respect and learn more about their lives, relationships, and communities—but they may be afraid of accidently saying the wrong thing and causing offense.

Using respectful language is a key way to communicate that you understand and accept an LGBT person's identity. Let's take a look at some key terminology:

LGBT: Generally speaking, the terms "lesbian," "gay," "bisexual," and "transgender" are considered respectful, and you should feel comfortable using the acronym "LGBT" as an umbrella word to speak about these people and communities.

Sexual orientation: "Lesbian," "gay," and "bisexual" (along with "straight" or "heterosexual") are words that describe a person's sexual orientation, or their emotional, intellectual, and physical attraction to other people.

Sex: The word "sex" describes a person's biological or physical characteristics, and most people are assigned the sex male or female at birth.

Gender: In everyday conservation people may use "sex" and "gender" interchangeably, but "gender" also includes all of the social and behavioral expectations that we associate with different sexes. Gender identity is how a person identifies, as either feminine, masculine, or according to a different gender identity. Gender identity is different from gender expression, which is how we all communicate our gender identity through clothing, voice, mannerisms, our names, and pronouns.

Transgender: The word "transgender" describes a person whose gender identity, or their internal and personal sense of their gender, is different than the sex they were assigned at birth. A transgender woman is someone who was assigned the sex male at birth but who identifies as a woman. The term "transgender man" describes someone who was assigned female at birth but is a man. The word "transgender" is an adjective, not a noun. You would say "transgender *person*," "transgender *woman*," or "transgender *man*"—not "a transgender" or "transgenders."

Cisgender: "Cisgender" is a word that describes a person whose gender identity aligns with the sex they were assigned at birth, for example, a person assigned male at birth and who identifies as a man.

Terms like "LGBT" are the most commonly used terms in the United States, but that means they also reflect the dominant European and Western cultural norms of this country, and some residents may not identify with these terms and instead use words that are specific to their racial, ethnic, or cultural heritage. For example, "Same Gender Loving" (SGL) is a term that some people use to describe their sexual orientation in a way that affirms the history of people of African descent. American Indian, Alaskan Native or Indigenous people may use the term "Two Spirit" to describe their identity. Some residents speak languages that do not have positive terms to describe LGBT identities, which means that discussing LGBT inclusion requires cultural as well as linguistic sensitivity.

There are several words that advocates recommend staff avoid when working with older adults. "Queer" has a long history of being used as a slur meant to harm LGBT people. In recent years the word "queer" has been reclaimed, meaning that people who identify in the LGBT spectrum have taken this historically negative term and made it into something positive. If you hear an older adult refer to themselves as "queer," you can ask if that is a word they would like others to use, or if it is a term that only they can use to describe their identity. Unless you know the resident identifies with the word "queer," I recommend avoiding it, even in a positive context, because it may trigger an older adult's traumatic associations or memories. Finally, you may hear people talk about "sexual preference" to describe attraction. I recommend that you use the term "sexual orientation" instead of "sexual preference," as the word "preference" suggests a person's attractions can be cured or changed.

As in many minority communities, there are some words that are acceptable for LGBT people to use when speaking to one another but which non-LGBT people should avoid. For example, you may hear a woman refer to herself or another woman as a "dyke." "Dyke," like "queer," is a word that can have positive or negative connotations. In this example, these women feel comfortable using that word but may be offended or alarmed if a man or non-LGBT person calls them "dykes." Since these words can have both positive and negative connotations, LGBT people may be more likely to trust that the intention is positive when it's coming from someone they perceive to be LGBT, but they won't be sure how to interpret it if it comes from someone else. Many of us are familiar with this "insider/outsider" dynamic and have experience navigating it in terms of race or ethnicity. You can apply the same sensitivities to working with LGBT people.

Some LGBT older adults may describe themselves using words that sound outdated or even offensive to younger LGBT people. For example, it is less common to use the word "trans-sexual" today as it often puts the focus on the medical aspects of the transgender experience, but older adults may identify with that term because it was the word that helped them make sense of their feelings when they came out. Likewise, people have varying reactions to the term "homosexual." Homosexuality was a diagnosable psychological disorder until 1973, and many people associate that term with negative medical experiences or the fear of being exposed or outed. Thus to them "homosexual" is an outdated and offensive term. Instead of the words "homosexual" or "homosexuality" you can say "gay," "lesbian," or "same-sex relationship." That said, for some older adults "homosexual" is the term they first used to understand their attractions and it may still make the most sense to them. If you hear a resident using a word that seems negative to you, your next step should be to have a conversation with the resident to determine if they are using the word in a positive or negative way.

These are general guidelines, and the important thing to remember is that each person will have their own understanding of these terms and their own preferences for how they describe their relationships and identity. The most important thing you can do is to not make assumptions about the words people use, and instead listen carefully and mirror back the language you hear. If a resident uses a term that you do not understand, it is perfectly OK to politely say something like, "That's a new word to me. Do you mind telling me what it means to you, and whether or not it's a word you'd like me and other residents to use?"

A HISTORY OF CHALLENGES AND SUCCESSES

We live in a rapidly changing world; the early 2000s and 2010s saw major advances in the rights of LGBT people. There are more LGBT people in the media and on television, marriage equality and the reversal of Don't Ask, Don't Tell have integrated LGBT people more fully into social institutions and civic life, and many more LGBT people live in states or communities with explicit non-discrimination protections.

When I tell people that a lot of LGBT older adults may be afraid to discuss their identities, people ask me, "If things are so much better today, why would someone be afraid to be open about their identity"?

To answer that question, we need to spend some time thinking about how an LGBT older person's experiences shape who they are and their sense of safety in the world. For example, in the 1950s lesbian and gay people were banned from federal employment, and thousands were fired for being, or being perceived to be, gay or lesbian. Homosexuality was a diagnosable psychological disorder until 1973, and transgender people are still diagnosed with a condition known as Gender Dysphoria. Consensual same-sex sexual activity between adults was illegal in some states until 2003, and many LGBT people still live in areas without explicit legal protections. Important advances in LGBT rights, like non-discrimination legislation and marriage equality, are relatively recent accomplishments.

BOX 1.2 ROB'S STORY

If I had to give advice to staff I'd say they need to understand the history of what it was like to be a gay man. I'm over 90 years old, and I came out when I was seventy, so I've seen a lot of changes. I grew up without any models of what it means to be a gay man. I went to the library and tried to learn about homosexuality, there was one book in the whole library, but it was a very general book and not what I was looking for or needed. I felt very isolated, and later I was struck that the American Psychiatric Association called homosexuality a mental disorder, and that wasn't changed until 1973. That change was not a scientific change; it was not based on new research, it was an ethical change. The ability to label something a sickness is a profound political power. A lot of the positive changes in acceptance that help me to feel comfortable being an openly gay man today are fairly recent, and I am not sure if younger people today realize that.

Rob

Many LGBT older adults have lived the majority of their lives in a world where their identities were seen as mental illness, criminal activity, or moral abomination. Later chapters in this book examine some of the health, financial, and psychological impacts of this history. Moreover, historical and present-day mistreatment around LGBT identity intersect with other aspects of people's identities too, and many LGBT people deal with dual realities of anti-LGBT bias compounded by things like racism, anti-Semitism, Islamophobia, ableism, and ageism, to name but a few. This has a real impact: as researchers have argued, "it is not being a sexual or gender minority or being an elderly person that is the main cause of social exclusion of LGBT elders; instead, it is the way in which society responds discriminately to them" (Harley, Gassaway, and Dunkley 2016, 564).

When someone is moving into your community they may feel vulnerable or nervous, especially if they are not choosing to make the move. Because they are in a more fragile state and navigating a new environment, going back into the closet often feels like the safest strategy until they have been assured that it is safe to be out. This book will give you some practical tools to help send that message of safety, but for now it is important to recognize that we are all shaped by our experiences, and many LGBT older adults have experienced a world where staying in the closet was a matter of life or death. Things are somewhat better today, but recent success does not mean that LGBT older adults will automatically feel safe or welcome in your community.

STRENGTH BASED IN HISTORY

LGBT older adults are a part of all of our communities, and while many face significant difficulties securing safe and supportive conditions for themselves, it is important to remember that these are resilient people. Having lived through a time when their identities were not accepted—sometimes even criminalized—many have come out the other side with a strong sense of self-reliance and a valuable set of experiences and perspectives. Staff play the key role in welcoming and supporting these people, and your LGBT community members may be some of your most dynamic. They have a lot to contribute once they know they can be themselves and feel confident that they will be treated with respect.

BOX 1.3   MY IDEAL RETIREMENT COMMUNITY

Some LGBT people prefer to live in communities specifically for LGBT older adults, while others prefer to live in general communities as long as they are safe and affirming. I asked SAGE participant and novelist Lujira Cooper to imagine her ideal retirement community:

> Gray Tigress Village, a community owned and operated by two women, was designed for maximum comfort of its older residents. Rooms painted in gold, teal, crimson, and off white had wide doors and efficiency kitchens. The expansive backyard contains violet lounging chairs, and sitting areas for conversation under shaded trees. Activities include bocce, tennis and basketball and a sparkling blue Olympic-sized pool dancing in the sunlight. Inside sits a spa with steam rooms and saunas surrounding another splendid pool. The food nutritious, delicious and plentiful. Desserts range from simple apple pie to decadent cheesecake.
>
> Nicknamed "tigress cove" by residents, it boasts a diverse clientele. Its tagline reads "come and meet women from everywhere." For older lesbians, it is home.

What strikes you about her description?

- Much of what she describes—good food, a pool and spa, bocce ball—would appeal to any potential resident.
- The community is owned by two women, meaning that the leadership reflects the clientele, who are also primarily women.
- There is diversity among the clientele, and the tagline explicitly describes it as a place for women from everywhere.
- The community's name projects strength and sensuality.

Chapter 2 explains in more detail what it means to come out, as well as some verbal and visual ways that you and your community can send a positive message to your current and future LGBT residents.

SUGGESTIONS

- Practice saying the acronym "LGBT" and the words "lesbian," "gay," "bisexual," and "transgender" so that you can say them without stumbling. Proceed with caution using the word "queer," and avoid terms like "homosexual" and "sexual preference."
- When in doubt, listen carefully and mirror back the terms and language the resident uses in conversation.
- Educate yourself and your staff about the historical events that shaped the lives of many LGBT people.
- Be sensitive to the fact that each person has lived their own journey, and that history impacts their sense of safety and willingness to be open about their identity and relationships.

FURTHER READING AND VIEWING

Diverse Elders Coalition (www.diverseelders.org)
Gen Silent (film) (www.theclowdergroup.com/gensilent).
"GLAAD Media Reference Guide—Terms to Avoid" (www.glaad.org/).
"Glosario de términos LGBT para equipos de atención a la salud" (www.lgbthealtheducation.org/).
"Inclusive Services for LGBT Older Adults: A Practical Guide to Creating Welcoming Agencies" (www.lgbtagingcenter.org/).
"LGBT Older Adults in Long-Term Care Facilities: Stories from the Field" (www.justiceinaging.org/).
"Maintaining Dignity: A Survey of LGBT Adults Age 45 and Older" (www.aarp.org/).

REFERENCES

Choi, Soon Kyu, and Ilan H. Meyer. 2016. "LGBT Aging: A Review of Research Findings, Needs, and Policy Implications." *The Williams Institute: UCLA School of Law.* https://williamsinstitute.law.ucla.edu/wp-content/uploads/LGBT-Aging-A-Review.pdf.

Espinoza, Robert. 2014. "Out and Visible: The Experiences and Attitudes of Lesbian, Gay, Bisexual and Transgender Older Adults, Ages 45–75." New York: SAGE. https://sageusa.org/files/LGBT_OAMarketResearch_Rpt.pdf.

Fredriksen-Goldsen, K.I. 2011. "Resilience and Disparities among Lesbian, Gay, Bisexual, and Transgender Older Adults." *Public Policy & Aging Report* 21 (3): 3–7. https://doi.org/10.1093/ppar/21.3.3.

Fredriksen-Goldsen, Karen I. 2016. "The Future of LGBT+ Aging: A Blueprint for Action in Services, Policies, and Research." *Generations (San Francisco, Calif.)* 40 (2): 6–15.

Fredriksen-Goldsen, Karen I., and Hyun-Jun Kim. 2017. "The Science of Conducting Research with LGBT Older Adults—An Introduction to Aging with Pride: National Health, Aging, and Sexuality/Gender Study (NHAS)." *The Gerontologist* 57 (suppl 1): S1–14. https://doi.org/10.1093/geront/gnw212.

Gates, Gary J. 2013. "LGBT Adult Immigrants in the United States." *The Williams Institute: UCLA School of Law.* https://williamsinstitute.law.ucla.edu/research/census-lgbt-demographics-studies/us-lgbt-immigrants-mar-2013/.

GLAAD. 2018. "Where We Are on TV Report—2018: GLAAD's Annual Report on LGBTQ Inclusion." *GLAAD.* www.glaad.org/whereweareontv18.

Harley, Debra A., Linda Gassaway, and Lisa Dunkley. 2016. "Isolation, Socialization, Recreation, and Inclusion of LGBT Elders." In *Handbook of LGBT Elders*, edited by Debra A. Harley and Pamela B. Teaster, 563–81. Cham: Springer International Publishing. https://doi.org/10.1007/978-3-319-03623-6.

Justice in Aging, National Gay and Lesbian Task Force, SAGE, Lambda Legal, National Center for Lesbian Rights, and National Center for Transgender Equality. 2015. "LGBT Older Adults in Long-Term Care Facilities: Stories from the Field." *Justice in Aging.* www.justiceinaging.org.customers.tigertech.net/wp-content/uploads/2015/06/Stories-from-the-Field.pdf.

Kim, Hyun Jun, Katherine Acey, Aundaray Guess, Sarah Jen, and Karen I. Fredriksen-Goldsen. 2016. "A Collaboration for Health and Wellness." *Generations* 40 (2): 49–55.

Kim, Hyun-Jun, Karen I. Fredriksen-Goldsen, Amanda E. B. Bryan, and Anna Muraco. 2017. "Social Network Types and Mental Health among LGBT Older Adults." *The Gerontologist* 57 (suppl 1): S84–94. https://doi.org/10.1093/geront/gnw169.

Kim, Hyun-Jun, Sarah Jen, and Karen I. Fredriksen-Goldsen. 2017. "Race/Ethnicity and Health-Related Quality of Life Among LGBT Older Adults." *The Gerontologist* 57 (suppl 1): S30–39. https://doi.org/10.1093/geront/gnw172.

Meyer, Ilan H., Soon Kyu Choi, and Krystal Kittle. 2018. "Aging LGB Adults in California: Findings from the 2015–2016 California Health Interview Survey." *The Williams Institute: UCLA School of Law.* https://williamsinstitute.law.ucla.edu/wp-content/uploads/1809-CHIS-Older-Adults-Report.pdf

Robinson-Wood, Tracy, and Amanda Weber. 2016. "Deconstructing Multiple Oppressions Among LGBT Older Adults." In *Handbook of LGBT Elders*, edited by Debra A. Harley and Pamela B. Teaster, 65–81. Cham: Springer International Publishing. https://doi.org/10.1007/978-3-319-03623-6.

Schwinn, Susan V., and Shirley A. Dinkel. 2015. "Changing the Culture of Long-Term Care: Combating Heterosexism." *Online Journal of Issues in Nursing* 20 (2): 7.

U.S. Census Bureau. n.d. "U.S. Census Bureau QuickFacts: Chicago City, Illinois." *U.S. Census Bureau.* Accessed February 16, 2018. www.census.gov/quickfacts/fact/table/chicago cityillinois/PST045216.

FIRST IMPRESSIONS

SUMMARY

This chapter discusses what it means to come out, the fact that LGBT people come out many times over their lives, and the ways in which LGBT people listen and look for cues that they will be safe and treated with respect. It emphasizes the importance of not making assumptions when meeting a new resident or potential resident and in everyday conversation. Finally, I look at how to make publicity materials and programming more attractive to current and future LGBT residents.

OBJECTIVES

- Understand what it means to "come out" as LGBT.
- Identify and learn to avoid words, phrases, or interview styles that may communicate assumptions about a person's sexual orientation or gender identity.
- Incorporate open-ended and LGBT-affirming conversational techniques and interview questions into your daily interactions with current and potential residents.
- Learn ways to make programming and publicity materials more attractive to LGBT residents.

COMING OUT OF THE CLOSET

Colloquially, when we say that someone is "coming out of the closet" or "coming out" we mean that this person is openly self-identifying as a member of the LGBT community. Sometimes this process is referred to as "self-disclosure." To say that someone is "closeted" or "in the closet" means that they are not openly disclosing their identity, and may be actively hiding it. Being "outed" is to have that identity disclosed by someone else, often against the wishes of the LGBT person.

Movies and television would have us believe that an LGBT person only comes out once, often in a stressful and dramatic moment. While it is true that coming out to close friends or family can be a particularly impactful and memorable event, the fact is that LGBT people come out hundreds if not thousands of times throughout their lives. For example, I came out to my family members when I was in college, and it was, indeed, a significant moment for me. But I also continue to come out every time I meet someone new and introduce them to my male partner, discuss my experiences as a gay man, or use phrases like "my community" when talking about LGBT people.

A person's LGBT identity may also be communicated by their clothing, mannerisms, voice, vocabulary, or any of the other things that make up our gender expression. Transgender people may be outed if their gender expression does not meet societal expectations, if their identity documents have different or incorrect names and gender markers, or if they are asked or required to remove their clothing.

The decision to come out, especially in a new setting like a long-term care or senior living community, requires that the LGBT person consider a number of concerns that can be grouped into the categories Who, What, Where, When, and Why:

- **Who** is the resident coming out to? Is the person they are speaking with LGBT themselves, or do they seem friendly and comfortable with LGBT people?
- **What** can be said? Do people in the community discuss LGBT issues or identities, or is the topic taboo? Is the discussion respectful or insulting?
- **Where** is the conversation happening? Is it in a private office or a common area? Are there other LGBT residents or staff present? How are they treated? Are there any images of LGBT people or symbols in the community? Is it clear that the community expects LGBT people to be treated with respect, and if so, is that expectation an explicit part of resident agreements or policies?
- **When** should a person come out? If they have been in the closet for years, does it feel like it will be too late? What are the risks of coming out right away?
- **Why** is the resident coming out? Do they feel pressured? Is it something they want to do, or are they being outed against their will?

This list is not exhaustive, but these are some of the things that, in conjunction with a person's personal history, may inform their decision about whether to come out.

Even if you yourself are not LGBT, I am sure you have experienced disclosing something personal and sensitive to someone else. Think of a time when you told someone something private. Perhaps it was about a family member's struggle with substance use, your own journey with depression or anxiety, or a painful or traumatic experience. In the moments before you tell someone this information, you may worry about their reaction and if it will change their perception of you or affect your relationship. It's a similar set of worries and calculations when coming out as LGBT. To be clear, coming out is not shameful or negative, but it does bring up specific worries about how the listener will respond and if it will change your relationship.

As staff it is important to create spaces where residents can come out if they choose to, without pressuring them to do so. As an advocate who is concerned with making people feel safe enough to come out, sometimes I need to remind myself that people have good reasons to decide to stay private about their identity. Indeed, overly emphasizing that people should come out can reflect an individualistic or Eurocentric mentality—which is to say, it can reflect assumptions about identities and relationships that are true in certain cultural contexts but may not be true for residents with other backgrounds. For LGBT older adults who live in rural areas or are people of color, members of immigrant communities, or from cultural or religious contexts that place special importance on familial cohesion over and above individualism and independence, the potential disruption and strain on these relationships caused by coming out could outweigh the personal desire to come out. This is especially true if family members are the primary caregivers for the LGBT older adult. In such situations, changing their relationship with their family could be detrimental. While it is essential to create a safe and welcoming space for residents to come out if they choose, many people have very good reasons not to come out and that decision should also be respected. For more information on how a person's identity and community may influence their ability and desire to come out see Chapters 6–15 of Harley and Teaster 2016.

If you think one of your residents is LGBT but they have not come out to you explicitly, you may wonder if it is OK to ask them directly. Generally speaking, it is not a good idea to ask this question directly. It may be perceived as invasive or threatening and increase the resident's stress and fear. Instead, this chapter and the next will explore how to send an affirming message that it is safe to be out, without explicitly asking residents if they are LGBT.

MEETING AND GREETING

What are the first questions you ask a prospective resident when they are touring your community or being discharged from the hospital into your care? What do you ask a new resident in order to start building a relationship and get to know them? Often these questions center around key life events and relationships, with questions like "Are you married?" or "Do you have kids or grandkids?" Even if you don't lead with these questions, many people assume that they can know a person's gender identity based on how they are dressed, their physical features, such as facial hair, or the tone and tenor of their voice. Staff may also assume that an older man and woman are married, or that a younger person accompanying a resident is their child.

But these assumptions might be wrong, and voicing them can send the message that the questioner thinks the resident is heterosexual and/or cisgender. One of the most important ways we can begin to create a more inclusive community is to identify how these assumptions influence the way we do our jobs and work to change them. Let's look at two different scenarios.

Asking for the restroom

Tom is at the reception desk and is busy with some filing. While he's looking at something in the filing cabinet he hears someone with a slightly lower voice say, "Excuse me, can you tell me where I can find the restroom?" Without looking up Tom replies, "The men's room is down the hall on the right." After a pause he looks up to see a woman standing at the reception desk looking startled and offended. She leaves without saying anything more.

Meeting with the sales director

Jane is the sales director. She's meeting with a woman who is looking to move into the community, and this woman arrives for the tour with two men who appear to be in their mid-40s. After shaking hands, all four people sit down to chat. As everyone is getting settled Jane turns to one of the men and asks, "Would you and your brother like some coffee?" The men exchange a look, and the rest of the conversation is stilted and uncomfortable.

Both of these examples show how a simple and common assumption can send the wrong message. In the first scenario the receptionist assumes that all people with deeper voices identify as men, which may make this woman feel uncomfortable and misunderstood. In the second, Jane assumes that the two men are bothers, when in fact one man is the woman's son and the other is his husband

It is easy to avoid these negative interactions. The receptionist could say something like, "All the bathrooms are down this hall to the right" and also mention if there is a gender-neutral or single-stall bathroom. The sales director can make it a point to only refer to people by their names until it becomes clear how they are related to one another.

The goal is not perfection, and we all make assumptions every day. The trick is to catch yourself before acting on an assumption. The following are some of the most common assumptions I see in senior residential settings:

- That a man and a woman are a couple.
- That two men or two women are family or friends and *not* a couple.
- That anyone with children or grandchildren is heterosexual and/or cisgender.
- That gay men are effeminate, that lesbian women are masculine, and that you can know if someone is transgender based on their physical appearance.
- That a younger person accompanying or visiting a resident is that person's child or grandchild.

It is important to be aware of these very common ways in which we all may accidently communicate that we think someone is straight and/or cisgender. At the same time, you need not become paranoid or afraid of accidentally causing offense. Most of these errors can be avoided by being aware of the many ways people identify and the kinds of relationships they might have. The most important thing you can do is be polite, listen carefully to how people talk about themselves and their relationships, and then reflect or mirror that language back.

OPEN-ENDED QUESTIONS: EVERY PROFESSIONAL'S BEST FRIEND

In addition to being more aware of our assumptions, it is important to recognize that many LGBT people have families or support structures that look different than the traditional nuclear family. The picture of a family with a mother, father, and two children does not often fit the LGBT community. It is quite common for people to come out later in life, perhaps after their children move away, their spouse dies, or they retire. Sometimes when they come out their children or other family members do not accept their identity and cut off all contact with the LGBT person. Other people may never have partnered or had children.

Being abandoned by family is a traumatic experience, and with older adults it is particularly scary because it is often family members who visit, provide informal care, help with housework and shopping, and otherwise make sure that older adults are doing OK. This is called a "vertical care network," where people of multiple ages and generations provide care for one another. LGBT older adults, especially those who have strained or no relationships with their biological or legal family members, tend to rely on what are called "chosen families" or "families of choice." These are often horizontal networks, where people provide care and support for others in their same age cohort. All of this means that LGBT older adults often rely on one another for support, and LGBT people are more likely to be caregivers. A recent study found that 20.4 percent of LGBT people are providing care for another person, compared to 16.5 percent of non-LGBT people (National Alliance for Caregiving 2015, 14).

I discuss navigating LGBT family dynamics in more depth in Chapter 7, but in terms of first impressions it is important that you ask questions that create an opening for residents to describe their chosen family. If you ask an LGBT resident, "Do you have any family?" the answer might be a flat "No," because to the resident the word "family" means biological family. However, if you ask questions that help to get a sense of their horizontal care network, their family of choice, you may get a fuller picture of that person's situation. Here are some open-ended questions to try:

- Who are the most important people in your life?
- Who would you call in an emergency?
- Who do you spend a lot of time with?
- Who would you call just to chat and catch up?
- Tell me about yourself.

The next step is to listen closely to what the resident tells you. LGBT older adults may hide the nature of their relationships or use euphemisms until they know they are safe. For example, an older lesbian woman might refer to her girlfriend as her "roommate," "friend," "sister," or "cousin."

If you think that a resident's "friend" might in fact be their partner or significant other, do not ask explicitly if they are. Simply refer to the person as their "friend" and see if later on, after you have developed a relationship, they tell you something new or give you more details about the nature of their relationship. Whenever you hear a resident mention someone several times, consider asking open-ended question like, "How long have you known so-and-so? She seems really great." The key is to affirm the relationship and ask for more information in a gentle way.

Staff should use these conversational techniques in all interactions with every resident, and you should make your programming LGBT-inclusive even if you do not think you have any LGBT community members. You cannot tell if someone is LGBT by looking at them, so being consistent is the best way to ensure that you are sending the right message to people who may be in the closet.

AFTER SOMEONE COMES OUT

If a resident tells you that they are LGBT, it is important to recognize that the conversation may have been stressful or scary. Thank them for their trust, and ask if they feel comfortable with you sharing that information with other staff or if they would prefer that you keep it private. You should never out anyone without their permission and should only break this confidence if you think that the resident is in danger. The fact that a resident is LGBT may not seem like a big deal to you, and you may know that other staff will be OK with it too, but you must always respect that the LGBT person has the right to control who does and does not know about their identity (The Joint Commission 2011, 27).

If you think that information about a person's LGBT identity should be entered into their file or case notes—for example, noting their partner's name, or the name and pronouns that they use—ask the resident if they feel comfortable having that information written down. A good rule of thumb is that you want to partner with the resident to make sure they feel safe and in control, not make decisions for them about who knows that they are LGBT.

PROGRAMMING AND OUTREACH MATERIALS

So far, I have discussed how to create a welcoming space in conversation with an LGBT older adult, but things like the images and language you use in advertisements, programming, and communications can also send a positive or negative message.

For example, many long-term care communities only have pictures of white, different-sex couples on their website, and those couples often present very standard masculine and feminine gender expressions. LGBT people scan their environments for cues that they will or will not be accepted. Including pictures of diverse LGBT people and families in advertisements is a good way to signal that LGBT people are welcome in your community. The rainbow flag and pink triangle are two of the most recognizable symbols for the LGBT community. The rainbow flag was created by San Francisco artist and activist Gilbert Baker in the late 1970s. There are several theories for why he chose the rainbow (including its association with gay icon Judy Garland's character, Dorothy, from *The Wizard of Oz*) but today it is recognized as a symbol of the LGBT community (Grovier n.d.). The pink triangle has a darker past. During the Nazi regime, between 5,000 and 15,000 gay men were sent to concentration camps and forced to wear the pink triangle on their clothing, similar to the yellow Star of David worn by Jewish people in concentration camps. This symbol has been reclaimed by LGBT people and is now a positive symbol affirming the community (Ziv 2015).

There are two approaches to LGBT programming. One option is to create programming specifically about or geared toward the LGBT community. This could be an LGBT movie and discussion, a support group for LGBT people, a Gender and Sexuality Alliance (GSA), or a social event celebrating Pride Month (typically June). The other option is to make sure that all of your existing programming is open to LGBT people. Ask yourself, are there places where you can make language more neutral or explicitly mention that LGBT people would be welcome? For example, imagine you are organizing a family picnic where residents and their families have lunch together. LGBT residents may not feel comfortable bringing their chosen family members and assume that this event is not for them. Changing the language to say, "A picnic for family, friends, and loved ones—everyone welcome!" can send a much more inclusive message and encourage LGBT residents to bring whomever they like to the event. I typically recommend that staff begin making existing programming more inclusive, while also laying the groundwork to start LGBT-specific programming. That being said, some communities may have a longer road ahead of them to LGBT-specific content, while others may be in a place to jump right in. Chapter 4 offers a more detailed discussion about how to create and edit programming for LGBT residents.

Finally, organizational standards and policies are another opportunity to send an affirming message. Many communities have a non-discrimination policy. Review that information to make sure the policy includes "sexual orientation, gender identity, and gender expression" as protected categories, and that all prospective and current residents read and understand those protections. These policies are often written in legal-sounding language and buried deep in the resident agreement. But they need not be. I have worked with communities to rewrite their policies so that they are more readable statements that can be front and center on community websites and in new resident information packets.

BOX 2.1   *DOR L'DOR*: GENERATION TO GENERATION

As I stood graveside and addressed the family gathered to escort their mother/grandmother's body to its final resting place, I noticed one of the deceased's grandsons was wearing a rainbow pin. Those of us who identify as LGBT+ tend to notice signs of LGBT+ affirmation, inclusion, celebration. I continued with the service.

After it ended, I approached the grandson and told him that I liked his rainbow pin. "My grandmother gave it to me," he said. "She attended a Pride Shabbat that you led at the Abramson Center for Jewish Life." That was not the response I was expecting. To hear that his almost 95-year-old grandmother was aware of the Pride Shabbat service and its meaning surprised me because of the state of her decline at that time.

I learned that his grandmother had enthusiastically shared with him details of the Pride Shabbat service and wore the pin on a beloved hat in solidarity with him, her precious grandson who is gay. Upon her death, he took the pin, now a treasured possession connecting him to his loving grandmother.

When you're working with elderly people in a long-term care facility you often don't see the broader "ripple" effect of your work, but in this instance, only a little over one month after our Pride Shabbat, I learned about a beautiful connection our LGBT+ Initiatives facilitated. I saw firsthand how our work not only benefits people directly in the LGBT+ community but also their loved ones and how it can foster stronger, deeper connections and understanding among people in unforeseen ways.

Rabbi Erica Steelman, MAHL, MPP
Director of LGBT+ Initiatives, Staff Chaplain
Abramson Center for Jewish Life

Everything described in this chapter will help to attract new LGBT residents and to send the message to current residents that they can come out of the closet, if they should choose to do so. One note of caution is that these symbols and signs of inclusion must be backed up by a staff that is prepared and willing to support LGBT residents. If you put a rainbow flag on your reception desk but your community is not in fact a safe place to be LGBT, you are setting a trap where someone might come out but not be safe. These visuals create a sense of safety, but they are only one of many components that create communities where LGBT older adults will find respect and acceptance.

BOX 2.2   MARIA ROBERTS' STORY

At our senior living community, one of our evening lecture series featured residents who are parents of LGBT children sharing their experience, and I was one of the presenters. The lecture was extremely well received with many favorable comments. Our son knows about the lecture, though he lives far away and was not present. Although he felt comfortable visiting us before Asbury adopted its welcoming policy, I know it is gratifying to him that his parents live in a welcoming community.

Maria Roberts
Resident of Asbury Methodist Village, Gaithersburg, MD

SUGGESTIONS

- Try not to make judgements or assumptions about people's sexual orientation or gender identity.
- Use gender-neutral and inclusive language on advertisements, applications, and promotional materials.
- Ask open-ended questions and listen for responses that invite more questions.
- Once staff have been trained and your policies are in place, use images like a rainbow flag and pictures of LGBT people and families on your website.
- Highlight your LGBT programming and audit your existing programming to make them more explicitly inclusive.

FURTHER READING AND VIEWING

"A Resource Guide to Coming Out" (www.hrc.org/).
"Resources for Coming Out Later in Life" (www.lgbtagingcenter.org/).
"Sexual Orientation and Gender Identity, Tip Sheet for the Preferences for Everyday Living Inventory (PELI)" (https://preferencebasedliving.com/).

REFERENCES

Grovier, Kelly. n.d. "The History of the Rainbow Flag." *BBC*. Accessed February 18, 2018. www.bbc.com/culture/story/20160615-the-history-of-the-rainbow-flag.
Harley, Debra A., and Pamela B. Teaster, eds. 2016. *Handbook of LGBT Elders*. Cham: Springer International Publishing. https://doi.org/10.1007/978-3-319-03623-6.

The Joint Commission. 2011. "Advancing Effective Communication, Cultural Competence, and Patient- and Family-Centered Care for the Lesbian, Gay, Bisexual, and Transgender (LGBT) Community." *The Joint Commission.* www.jointcommission.org/assets/1/18/LGBTFieldGuide_WEB_LINKED_VER.pdf.

National Alliance for Caregiving. 2015. "Caregiving in the U.S., 2015 Report." *AARP.* www.aarp.org/content/dam/aarp/ppi/2015/caregiving-in-the-united-states-2015-report-revised.pdf.

Ziv, Stav. 2015. "Pink Triangles and Prison Sentences: Nazi Persecution of Homosexuals." *Newsweek.* May 31, 2015. www.newsweek.com/pink-triangles-prison-sentences-nazi-persecution-homosexuals-337840.

MOVE-IN DAY AND COLLECTING INFORMATION

3

SUMMARY

This chapter outlines ways to create a smooth move-in process for new LGBT residents, including how to collect information on residents' sexual orientation and gender identity, how staff can respectfully ask someone about their sexual orientation and gender identity, when it is appropriate to ask these questions, when they should not be asked, and responses to common pushback or concerns from both staff and residents.

OBJECTIVES

- Learn why collecting information on a resident's sexual orientation and gender identity is a vital part of providing person-centered care.
- Examine example questions related to sexual orientation and gender identity, as well as responses to common pushback.
- Learn when it is, and is not, appropriate to ask these questions.
- Consider the fact that we all have sexual orientations and gender identities, and they play a crucial role in all of our lives.

MOVING IN

The big day is here! The paperwork has been signed, the boxes are packed, and your staff are welcoming the newest resident or residents to your community. Moving is always stressful, and while some residents may be thrilled to start their new lives in your community, others may not be happy to be leaving their homes, may be dealing with complicated medical conditions, or may be fearful about fitting in with their new neighbors. With all the hectic activity, a new resident's sexual orientation or gender identity may be the last thing on a staff person's mind, and if the question is brought up they may say, "Why is it any of my business if a resident is LGBT?"

Many older adults may feel perfectly comfortable talking about their identity but choose not to do so because they consider it private information. That is their right and it should be respected; but consider the perspective of someone who does want to be open but is unsure or scared about how they will be treated if they come out. A bisexual woman may not feel comfortable discussing her long-term relationship with a female partner who passed away last year. A transgender man could be afraid to dress in clothes that reflect his gender identity or not feel comfortable talking about his childhood. A gay man might feel pressure to hide pictures of his boyfriend, or throw them away before moving into your community. For these reasons it is important to remember that being LGBT is about more than sex and gender—it is about a resident's personal history and their friends, family, and community.

In Chapter 2, I described ways of using visuals such as rainbow flags and LGBT-inclusive photographs to send a message that LGBT people are welcome in the community, and I offered suggestions for how to have open-ended conversations. In this chapter I want to discuss how and when it is appropriate to ask a resident directly about their sexual orientation and gender identity, and how that information can be recorded and used to help staff.

WHY DO WE NEED TO KNOW?

LGBT advocates have long argued that we need intake tools and census forms that collect information on a person's sexual orientation (SO) and gender identity (GI) (these questions are often referred to as "SOGI questions," pronounced SOH-jee).

The need for this information is summed up in the phrase "If you're not counted, you don't count!" For example, the 2010 United States census did not have any explicit questions about sexual orientation or gender identity. Respondents could say if they were living with a same-sex spouse or same-sex unmarried partner, which allowed statisticians to get a broad picture of where some LGBT people live, but it did not count single lesbian, gay, and bisexual people, bisexual people in different-sex relationships, or many transgender people.

Similarly, very few aging service providers or surveys for older adults include SOGI questions. Those that do may find it difficult to get LGBT people to answer these questions because they are afraid of coming out to a provider or stranger on the phone. Without this information we cannot know the population's size, health, financial status, psychological wellbeing, or other specific information about LGBT older adults, making it more difficult to advocate for increased funding for programs that help LGBT people.

Within a senior living community, this information is essential to answering a number of important questions: Do you have LGBT residents? Do they have any specific needs or concerns? How are they enjoying your community? Do they feel welcome, and are your efforts to become more LGBT-inclusive having an impact on your residents' wellbeing?

There are, however, advocates who do not think that questions about sexual orientation and gender identity should be added to intake forms. Some fear that recording that information might make LGBT people more vulnerable to staff or other residents who are anti-LGBT. One report that surveyed over 4,000 LGBT people and people living with HIV of many ages found that more than half of respondents had experienced some form of discrimination in healthcare, with higher rates among people of color and transgender and gender-nonconforming people (Lambda Legal 2010). Disclosing an LGBT identity or HIV status can lead to better care, but it can make someone more vulnerable to abuse.

Others argue that asking these questions, especially during what is a politically divisive time in our nation, may make LGBT older people more fearful and more likely to go back into the closet. These are very real concerns. If you are working in a setting where LGBT people are vulnerable, and if you do not think other staff members will treat LGBT residents with respect, consider not asking these questions until you can establish training and policies that will protect residents if they do decide to come out.

Assuming that your organization is already implementing or has decided to begin implementing LGBT-inclusive questions during the move-in process, let's consider some best practices for making these questions an opportunity for affirmative self-disclosure, rather than a scary or awkward conversation.

WHEN AND HOW TO ASK SOGI QUESTIONS

Staff have various points of contact with residents during the move-in process. From the first visit to the tour, collecting paperwork and medical records, all the way to move-in day, when is the right time to ask a resident about their LGBT identity?

As a general rule of thumb, SOGI questions can be incorporated into any private setting where you are asking for other potentially sensitive demographic information, such as information about a person's race, ethnicity, religion, medical history, and questions about mental health or income. It should always be clear that these questions are optional and can be skipped if the resident chooses.

You should not ask SOGI questions in a setting where that information could be used to discriminate or influence a decision-making process. For example, it is illegal for a hiring manager to ask a job candidate about their race or religion. While not all states have job discrimination protections for LGBT people, you should avoid asking SOGI questions in these settings. Likewise, these questions are inappropriate to ask a potential resident or someone who is not currently using your services, because asking these questions at that time could introduce prejudice in the application, admissions, or decision-making process.

Another strategy is to let people complete this information at home as a part of their welcome packet because residents may be more forthright about their identity and experiences when completing a survey at home (Alper, Feit, and Sanders 2013).

A SOGI question that only asks, "Do you identify as LGBT?" is not sufficient. While this question will tell your staff if someone considers themselves a part of the LGBT community, it does not give you detailed enough information about how they identify, or in what way they consider themselves part of the LGBT community. That is because everyone has both a sexual orientation and gender identity. If a resident tells you that they are gay, then you have learned about their sexual orientation, but you have not learned anything about their gender identity. Likewise, a resident can tell you that they are transgender—providing information about their gender identity—but that does not tell you anything about their sexual orientation. Some transgender people may not be public about the fact that they are transgender; they simply say that they are a man or woman. In this instance, it is best to have a question that affirms their gender identity while also creating space for them to tell you they are a person of transgender experience. We all have both a sexual orientation and gender identity, and a well-crafted set of SOGI questions will provide the opportunity for residents to tell you about both aspects of their identity.

That is why it is a best practice to have at least two questions: one allowing for a person to describe their sexual orientation and another to capture gender identity and whether they identify as transgender.

BOX 3.1   SAMPLE SOGI QUESTIONS

The following questions are from a guide titled *Inclusive Questions for Older Adults: A Practical Guide to Collecting Data on Sexual Orientation and Gender Identity*, produced by the National Resource Center on LGBT Aging (French 2016). There are many other ways to ask these questions, so please consider researching other suggestions to see what works best for your community and your staff.

Sexual orientation

Do you think of yourself as . . .

a) Heterosexual or straight
b) Lesbian or gay
c) Bisexual
d) Not listed above, please specify _____
e) Not sure
f) Decline to answer

This question allows a series of responses but also provides the opportunity for someone to decline to answer, provide their own answer, or invite more conversation by stating that they are not sure.

Gender identity

What is your current gender identity (choose ALL that apply)?

a) Male
b) Female
c) Female-to-Male (FTM)/Transgender Male/Trans Man
d) Male-to-Female (MTF)/Transgender Female/Trans Woman
e) Not listed above: Please specify _____
f) Decline to Answer

What sex were you assigned at birth on your original birth certificate (Check one)?

a) Male
b) Female
c) Decline to Answer

This two-part question allows the resident to note their current gender identity, which tells you and your staff how they wish to be identified. It also collects data on their sex assigned at birth. This gives the resident the ability to identify as Male or Female (and not explicitly as transgender), while also signaling to you that they are a person of transgender experience which may be important information when processing their documents or organizing personal or medical care.

Additionally, a question like "What pronouns do you use? For example, he/him, she/her, they/them" can create an opportunity to let the resident tell you their pronouns. Chapter 10 has more information on the importance of correct names and pronouns.

Finally, consider translating forms into other languages if that will make the interviewee more comfortable. You can find sample questions translated into Traditional Chinese, Spanish, Filipino, Vietnamese, and Russian at the National Resource Center on LGBT Aging's website (lgbtagingcenter.org).

Many electronic medical record programs do not allow for anything other than a binary (M/F) question related to sex, and certain reimbursements, such as those for Medicare and Medicaid, may also require reporting on forms that only have binary options. It may not be possible to change those forms and electronic medical records controlled by the government or private companies. If that is the case, you can make more robust notes about a person's identity in the Notes or Narrative field of their record. If you do need to mark down a sex that does not align with the resident's identity, perhaps for the purposes of insurance or reimbursement, it is best to explain why this is necessary and obtain the resident's permission. You may say something like, "I know and respect who you are, and in order to make sure this claim is processed correctly, it might be best to enter the sex you were assigned at birth. Are you OK with me doing that?" Collecting SOGI information is a relatively new practice across aging service providers, so your organization may need to be creative when interfacing with government requirements and electronic medical records while also storing and communicating this information in a safe and effective way.

This information should be kept strictly confidential.

Setting the stage

Like all potentially sensitive questions, it is not a good idea to start off a conversation with SOGI questions. Take some time to get to know the resident, introduce yourself, chat about the weather or your community, and start to build rapport. Another good way to set the right tone is to begin by reading the community's LGBT-inclusive nondiscrimination policy, and explaining that all residents are welcome. Similarly, casually walking through some of the LGBT-inclusive programming in your community can help make it clear that you are LGBT-welcoming. For example, "We host a Japanese cooking hour, murder mystery book club, some of our residents participate in LGBT Pride every year, which is coming up soon, and we offer tons of other field trips!" This casually informs the resident that there are already LGBT people or allies in the community and may help them feel more comfortable answering SOGI questions later in your conversation.

Before asking demographic questions, including SOGI questions, make it clear that all of the questions are optional, the resident can skip any question they do not want to answer, and they can change their answers in the future. This can help ensure that a resident does not feel pressured to answer a question that may be a surprise or initially uncomfortable. The resident may decline to answer these questions but then return to change their answer once they are more comfortable with the staff and their neighbors. You can also provide these questions beforehand in the welcome packet, giving the resident the opportunity to answer them in private.

Finally, make the questions boring! Asking SOGI questions may feel scary or embarrassing at first, but like anything, practice makes perfect. Work with a colleague to practice asking the question so that you can say it naturally, in an even tone of voice. Keep body language neutral and behave as though these questions are the most boring questions in the world. Residents will pick up on your discomfort or nerves, so keeping things calm is important to making the conversation comfortable.

Personal preference worksheets

Another time to provide opportunities to come out is when staff are collecting information about a person's personal history, interests, and preferences. Many communities have a "Getting to Know You" worksheet or set of interview questions that cover things like when a person likes to get up and shower, what their interests are, how they like to dress, personal grooming regimens, food likes and dislikes, etc. There is a version of the Preferences for Everyday Living Inventory (PELI) called the Rainbow PELI (2017) that has edited many of the questions to be more inclusive.

BOX 3.2   THE RAINBOW PELI (PREFERENCES FOR EVERYDAY LIVING INVENTORY)

The following are two questions taken from the Rainbow PELI ("Preferences for Everyday Living Inventory (PELI)" 2017).

Question 1:
First Name: _____   Nickname: _____
Mr./Mrs./Ms./Dr.: _____   Other Name: _____

What pronoun would you like me to use when I greet you?

He, His, Him   She, Her, Hers   They, Them, Theirs Other: _____

The question above allows residents to tell you the name that they use, which may be different from the name that appears on their documents. Additionally, it allows you to capture the correct pronoun, with options that go beyond he/she.

What kind of club most interested you in the past?

Book club	Glee club
Crochet/knitting club	Card club
Computer club	Outdoors club
Church club	Religious club
Political club	Elks
VFW	American Legion
Red Hat Society	Music Club
LGBT Club	Movie Club
Exercise Club	Language Club
Gay-Straight Alliance	Arts Club
Drama Club	

Cultural/Ethnic club, please specify; _____
Support Group, please specify; _____
Other:_____

This question has two options, LGBT Club and Gay-Straight Alliance, that will allow a resident to signal that LGBT people and cultures are an interest, without explicitly coming out. It also demonstrates to someone who is trying to see if your community is a safe one that your staff know some residents have these interests and take the time to ask.

Seeing these possible responses sends the message that LGBT people are already living in and welcome in your community, and even if the resident does not come out (or if they are not LGBT), staff can discover if they are interested in being engaged in your LGBT programming and events or in conversation around the topic of LGBT politics.

BOX 3.3   WHY INCLUSIVE INTAKE IS KEY

We are senior service providers; why would we ask someone about their gender or sexual orientation?! How embarrassing!

It's true, given the norms over the past hundred years or so, it might feel a bit embarrassing. But embarrassing can be OK sometimes. It pales in comparison to the feeling of being invisible.

We know that some of the older adults who call to ask about services, as well as some of the clients in our programs, are transgender, gender fluid, or another gender identity. When only "male" and "female" are listed on intake forms, those folks are being told unequivocally that *their life is not an option*. Imagine that for a moment. Imagine if it happened over and over, across the course of your lifespan. That is how it's been for many of today's older LGBT adults.

The same, of course, holds true for sexual orientation, which is why all of our forms have LGBT-inclusive options, sending the message that these seniors are real, equal, and visible.

What if you ask these questions and you get a response like, "Why are you asking that?" or, "None of your business!"? This probably will happen, so it's good to be prepared! Simply and calmly answer that you and your agency are working towards equity for all. If they press, assure them everyone receives the exact same questions so that we know how to best serve each person. If possible, do the intakes in-person and have the client check their answers themselves, or send it to them beforehand.

Even if your agency has a reputation for being inclusive you *must* overtly signal your acceptance with a rainbow pin on your badge, or a welcoming emblem on your website, and a strong non-discrimination policy. Although you are fully accepting, older adults will still often hide unless you make these extra efforts. Even those who have lived their lives "out of the closet" might have retreated again as they have aged and grown more vulnerable. And no one should have to hide at any age, let alone in their older years.

We know not all of our participants will come out on these forms, but we trust that even seeing the inclusive options will make them feel seen and recognized as unique and valuable people!

Patricia Osage
Executive Director, LIFE ElderCare
Fremont, CA

Responding to pushback

While these questions may feel new, there are likely a number of personal questions about things like grooming, hygiene, personal history, religion, or income that staff are already used to asking. Think of SOGI questions in the same way as these initially awkward but now routine questions. That said, it is important to be prepared for a negative or confused response, such as

"Why are you asking me this?"
"None of your business!"
"Do I look gay to you?"

There are a number of ways to respond. First, emphasize that these questions are asked in all move-in conversations. This is important because the resident may think you are only asking these questions because you are curious or suspect that they are LGBT. Second, explain that the community is a diverse and welcoming place, and these questions are an important way for the community's staff to learn about residents and make sure they are responding to each resident's needs and preferences. Third, remind the resident that they can skip any question they like, and offer to move on. If the resident remains agitated or seems stuck on the question, it may be worth flagging to a supervisor to have a future conversation with the resident about why they reacted so strongly to the SOGI questions. It is one of the first opportunities to communicate your community's openness to LGBT residents and also to learn if other residents are uncomfortable or hostile to discussions of LGBT identity and may require some additional attention from staff to ensure they are comfortable with the community's expectations around mutual respect.

MOVE-IN DAY AND INTRODUCTIONS

Few things can start up the rumor mill faster than news of a new neighbor moving in, and staff have an important role to play in preparing the community to welcome all new residents. If a new LGBT resident is open about their identity with staff, it is appropriate to ask the resident if they have any concerns about moving in. Some people may not be worried at all, while others might be fearful about how their new neighbors will react. Let the resident guide your staff on whether they want the staff to have any preparatory conversations with other residents. They may want a staff member to tell other residents that a same-sex couple is moving in—for example, casually mentioning to residents that "John and Larry" are moving in soon—or to have some conversations about LGBT identities and culture. Others may prefer to be treated just like any new community member. What staff should avoid is accidentally contributing to the rumor mill by "warning" or "alerting" other residents that an LGBT person or persons is moving in. This makes being LGBT seem shameful or shocking. Staff should not disclose a new resident's sexual orientation, gender identity, or relationship status without that resident's consent. Any conversations with other residents should be respectful and in line with the wishes of new LGBT resident(s), and they should never disclose someone's LGBT identity without their permission.

If your community does not ask SOGI questions, it is important to review the suggestions in Chapter 2 about how to avoid assumptions and how to have open-ended conversations. Quality care is all about getting to know the person, and these questions combined with avoiding assumptions are important tools for getting to know your LGBT residents.

SUGGESTIONS

- LGBT-inclusive intake questions can be asked of all residents alongside other optional demographic information. The questions should always be optional.
- Use this data to get a picture of the specific interests, experiences, and needs of your LGBT residents. This data should be kept confidential.
- Make it clear that all residents are asked the same questions, and that nobody is being singled out for specific questions.
- Train staff on how to ask these questions before implementing any changes to intake forms or procedures.

FURTHER READING AND VIEWING

"Focus on Forms and Policy: Creating an Inclusive Environment for LGBT Patients" (www. lgbthealtheducation.org/).
"Inclusive Questions for Older Adults: A Practical Guide to Collecting Data on Sexual Orientation and Gender Identity" (www.lgbtagingcenter.org/).
"Ready, Set, Go! Guidelines and Tips for Collecting Patient Data on Sexual Orientation and Gender Identity (SO/GI)" (www.lgbthealtheducation.org/).

REFERENCES

Alper, Joe, Monica N. Feit, and Jon Q. Sanders. 2013. *Collecting Sexual Orientation and Gender Identity Data in Electronic Health Records: Workshop Summary*. Washington, D.C.: The National Academies Press.

French, Scott. 2016. "Inclusive Questions for Older Adults: A Practical Guide to Collecting Data on Sexual Orientation and Gender Identity." New York: The National Resource Center on LGBT Aging. www.lgbtagingcenter.org/resources/resource.cfm?r=601.

Lambda Legal. 2010. "When Health Care Isn't Caring: Lambda Legal's Survey of Discrimination Against LGBT People and People with HIV." New York: Lambda Legal. www.lambda legal.org/health-care-report.

Preference Based Living. "Preferences for Everyday Living Inventory (PELI) Nursing Home Version (Rainbow PELI-NH-Full)." 2017. *Preference Based Living*. https://preferencebasedliv ing.com/sites/default/files/PELIReportv3_Rainbow%20%281%29.pdf.

LGBT PROGRAMMING AND SERVICES

4

SUMMARY

What are the best ways to make LGBT-specific programming a part of your normal calendar of activities and services? Starting LGBT programming requires care and a thoughtful rollout to ensure it isn't rocky, under-attended, or controversial. In this chapter, we will explore several approaches to programming, common forms of pushback, and some ideas that can help inspire your team to start creating LGBT programming.

OBJECTIVES

■ Understand the pros and cons of programming specifically for LGBT residents, versus making all programming LGBT-inclusive.
■ Consider ways to advertise and promote programming that will not "out" or inadvertently marginalize LGBT residents.
■ Articulate responses to residents who are upset or offended by LGBT content.
■ Decide which approach to programming is the best place to start or to expand LGBT programming in your community.

TWO APPROACHES TO LGBT PROGRAMMING AND SERVICES

Creating programming and services explicitly for LGBT residents is an important way to support residents who are out and to set a positive and welcoming tone for residents who may be considering coming out. LGBT programming raises important questions. How will residents react? Will people who attend LGBT programming be marginalized? Which programming should be only for LGBT residents, and which should be open to all? There are at least two ways to increase your LGBT programming: creating LGBT-specific programming and ensuring all programming is open to all. Staff will need to determine if one approach is the best fit for your community at this time or if you will tackle both simultaneously.

Option one: Create LGBT-specific or themed programming

The first approach is to take the type of programming you are accustomed to and creating specifically LGBT versions of that programming. For example, in Box 4.1 the column on the left is programming typically seen in senior living and on the right is how it can be made LGBT-specific.

BOX 4.1   LGBT-SPECIFIC PROGRAMMING

General programming	LGBT-specific programming
Coffee and current events hour	Gender and sexuality in the news
Welcoming committee	LGBT inclusion subcommittee
Tax and legal affairs clinic	A meeting with lawyers specifically for LGBT families and tax concerns.
Movie night	Pride film festival during June
Visits to restaurants or community events	A group visit to the "gayborhood" or LGBT community space
Lectures or university classes	A lecture series on women's and gender studies, LGBT studies, or queer theory
Bingo or game night	Inviting a local drag queen or drag king to host "inclusion bingo"
Caregiver, grief, or other support group	A meeting that is only for LGBT people, LGBT caregivers, LGBT bereavement, etc.

At first you may consider making certain existing events or meetings about LGBT topics. For example, during Pride Month select an LGBT-themed movie. Adding an "LGBT spin" to an already successful program can help to test the waters and gauge interest and reactions to the topic. If that proves successful, then staff can consider creating dedicated programming, like a Gender and Sexuality Alliance (GSA).

BOX 4.2   STARTING A GSA OR GENDER AND SEXUALITY ALLIANCE

Originally called Gay-Straight Alliances, GSAs are clubs or groups that allow LGBT people and allies to meet one another, find support, and often organize or engage in activism. Today most people use the term Gender and Sexuality Alliance to be more inclusive of bisexual, transgender, and other people who do not identify as gay or straight but consider themselves a part of the LGBT community. Starting a GSA in your community can be a great way to create a space for residents to meet one another and raise LGBT issues and concerns, and it shows that LGBT inclusion is a routine part of your programming and community culture.

One decision that staff and residents will need to make is whether an event is exclusively for LGBT residents. This is most often the case if it is a support group or another event where identity plays a central role in the activity or the goal of the event. Just like a "women's worship group" or a bereavement group, these can be important spaces for people with a certain identity, or who share a particular experience, to come together and build community. These closed events should always be balanced with programming that addresses LGBT issues but is open to everyone in the community.

The advantage of specific programming that is explicitly about LGBT topics is that it sends a clear message that LGBT people are members of the community and there are safe spaces to meet and have fun. One risk is that other community members will think that anyone who attends these groups is LGBT, and closeted residents may feel too exposed or afraid to attend. To that end, with the exception of closed contexts like support groups, make it clear that anyone is welcome to attend these events, and encourage non-LGBT residents to attend in order to make the events seem unremarkable and to dispel the misperception that only LGBT people would be interested in participating.

Option two: Ensure all programming is open to LGBT people

The second approach does not entail creating new programming but instead focuses on ensuring that existing programming periodically discusses LGBT themes and is open to LGBT people. Similar to the suggestions in the previous section about adding LGBT content into existing programming, the goal here is that when LGBT topics arise in your existing programming the discussions are welcome and respectful.

For example, the programming team might not be ready to host an art exhibition focused on the work of LGBT artists or art emerging from the HIV/AIDS crises, but if the group is discussing the work of David Hockney they can mention that he is gay and discuss how that might influence his work. Or a community could show a film by Cheryl Dunye and discuss how her identity as a black lesbian influences her films. Some residents and staff might be inclined to "not go there" and keep that part of the artist's life and work hidden, so by being explicit and normalizing a discussion of the artists' intersectional identities, staff can help set an inclusive tone for the group. Again, the activity does not need to be explicitly LGBT, but the way the activity unfolds can either be welcoming or it can establish a negative "Don't Ask, Don't Tell" atmosphere. The goal should always be to make activities welcoming.

BOX 4.3 "WHAT DOES YOUR HUSBAND DO?"

"What does your husband do?" After years of working with older adults, this question and all it contains still rattles me. It assumes so much: Assumes I am in a relationship. Assumes the gender identity of the person I would be with. Assumes this theoretical partner's most important attribute is related to work. Assumes I even *want* to be in a relationship. As a mental health provider coming to work with older adults after working in a large forensic setting, I was unprepared for how often my appearance, identity, and relationships would be topics of conversation. Navigating these situations has been tricky but has also resulted in rich and inclusive community.

In assisted living, every move, every behavior is observed. I learned that the way I answered personal questions could be instrumental in signaling to older adult residents that I am a safe person to approach. In response to questions about the way I dressed, I made normalizing statements about inclusivity and identity and talked about all the different reasons people make choices around clothing, hair, and other aspects of appearance and presentation. I used myself as an example, and also opened up about changing fashions and social norms; these statements communicated to all in earshot that we did not need to conform to traditional gender norms in our interactions with each other.

Responding to personal questions and creating inclusive spaces is not easy. Neither is being out or totally open at work. Sometimes I felt myself wanting to do something shocking or challenging in response to assumptions about me. For example, when an out coworker told me one of the residents we worked with was telling people I "must be a lesbian because she always wears grey slacks" I reacted by telling my coworker I was going to wear a pink fluffy ballgown for the next week. We laughed about it, and I did not actually come to work dressed that way, but the impulse illustrates how easily these comments can push my buttons. In a reactive state, I fell right into a trap and perpetuated stereotypes in my response. I sometimes bite back sharp responses to the questions about husbands and children. There have been several situations where I have found myself code-switching, playing pronoun games, or deflecting questions and then reflecting back later, wishing I made different choices; it is a process. The more authentically I conduct myself in my work with older adults, the more space I can create for their own authentic expression.

For example, my early interactions with "Elizabeth" were about poetry; I did not realize right away that she was using poetry to vet me and my possible reactions to her identity. She spent her adulthood in creative communities in both New York and California, had a rich knowledge of poetry, and was connected to the feminist and lesbian poets of her era. In asking about my familiarity with these specific poets, she was seeing whether I could be trusted with her whole identity, her whole self. She asked if we could discuss some of their poems in our poetry group; I suggested she share the poems and I would share some about the lives of the poets. We could have discussed their poems without talking about their identities, but doing so would miss an opportunity to welcome the discussion of sexuality and gender into assisted living—topics often assumed to be off-limits or unwelcome. Bringing these poets and talking about their experiences and identities in our poetry group enabled Elizabeth to bring her own identity into the community. She eventually came out to me and talked about her long-term partner. Eventually, she felt safe enough to come out to the group and to mention her partner by name in conversations with other residents.

I am aware of the privilege of my position—I have fewer decades of stigma and bias to contend against in coming out. Older adults in care communities are also facing potential discrimination from those who provide care. I use the privilege I have to establish safe and inclusive group spaces and to communicate my openness to individuals. Doing so does not require disclosing my entire relationship history or a timeline of my identity formation, but it does require openness to discussing different topics in group settings, as I did with Elizabeth. By being myself at work, while still maintaining my privacy, I hope that other residents will also see me as an ally and a possible confidant.

Erin Partridge, PhD, ATR-BC
Elder Care Alliance

Similar to changes you can make to marketing materials, consider opportunities to make programming more gender-neutral and to change anything that may imply that the activity is only for non-LGBT residents. For example, if you are creating a flyer for a holiday dance or senior prom, rather than choosing clipart depicting a different-sex couple, use an image of music notes or tap shoes. You can also include specific language like, "Come dance with your spouse, partner, friends, or by yourself!" These changes make it clear that everyone is welcome, not just different-sex couples.

Consider if your activity rooms are gendered. For example, many communities have separate "arts and crafts" rooms that may be more feminine and "tool shop" spaces that are masculine. Even apart from LGBT inclusion, this could dissuade a man from taking a painting class and a woman from learning how to do carpentry. Calling the shared space a "studio" and using neutral colors and decorations make it more inviting for everyone.

Finally, wear a rainbow pin on your nametag, add a safe space poster to your office, mention an LGBT movie you saw over the weekend, or leave this book on a community book shelf! All of these subtle actions can express your openness to discussing LGBT concerns and your interest in LGBT inclusion.

These are only a handful of examples of how the activities your residents and staff already enjoy can become ways for a positive message to get out. Be creative, experiment, and see what works for you and your team.

MAINTAINING AN INTERSECTIONAL APPROACH

One thing I always have to remind myself is to not just focus on the LGBT side of things and try to create programming where people will not feel the need to choose between identities. For example, many LGBT people have had negative experiences with organized religion, and staff creating LGBT-affirming programming may, with good reason, avoid religious themes, discussions, or topics to ensure that LGBT residents feel welcome. This may work just fine for some LGBT elders who are not interested in religion, but many LGBT people identify closely with religious traditions. We know, for example, that 87 percent of African-Americans identify with some kind of religious affiliation, and an African-American LGBT resident may be very interested in programming that affirms their religious identity and spiritual needs (Sahgal and Smith 2009). Similarly, some of your LGBT residents may want to have a wine and cheese mixer for Pride, but others may be in recovery from alcoholism and find such an event alienating.

Not all LGBT people will feel equally welcome in an LGBT space. Bisexual and transgender people may not be interested in an LGBT space that seems to mostly focus on gay and lesbian experiences. LGBT people of color may not be comfortable in a space that is predominately white. Religious LGBT people may not want to discuss LGBT politics because they feel lumped in with anti-LGBT religious conservatives.

Do not let this overwhelm you—every group and every individual is unique and all programming requires being attentive to people's varied experiences. This is just a reminder that an LGBT space will not be automatically inviting and will not be experienced by everyone in the same way. No single event will satisfy every participant, but trying a multitude of ideas, surveying residents, and cultivating an intersectional approach to your programming will help make activities stronger and more popular.

RESPONDING TO PUSHBACK, RUMORS, AND SNICKERING

Adding LGBT programming to your calendars will definitely generate conversations with staff and residents!

A smooth rollout will benefit from doing some research ahead of time to gauge interest. One strategy is to poll residents about their ideas for new programming and include options or prompts that are LGBT-specific, like a discussion group, attending Pride, or a support group. Make the survey anonymous or a simple vote—that way staff can gauge interest in different ideas without future participants needing to out themselves. Anonymous feedback and survey tools are great ways to allow closeted or private residents to raise ideas and concerns.

If you are hosting programs that are only for LGBT people, residents may be curious about who is attending, and closeted residents may be afraid to attend because it will make it difficult for them to remain private about their identity. A GSA or a program about being an LGBT ally are good ways to start discussing LGBT inclusion and also make it clear that attendance does not mean that someone is LGBT. That being said, for programming that would out someone, such as a closed discussion group for people living with HIV/AIDS, consider asking interested participants when and where they would like to meet. Perhaps they can meet off-site, in a less heavily trafficked area, or at a time of day when residents are busy with meals or other programs. Staff should also be sensitive to not marginalize these programs or make them seem shameful. To balance these competing goals, try incorporating the participants into decisions about timing and venue. That way everyone involved will feel empowered.

Some residents may be upset with the new programming or the LGBT focus on an ongoing event. That is a good opportunity to have a one-on-one conversation to get more information and help them discuss their feelings and also build some awareness about LGBT people that could help change their mind.

BOX 4.4   RESPONSES TO COMMON PUSHBACK

Pushback	Sample response
Why would we have a GSA? There aren't any gay people here.	We can't make assumptions about other residents, and even if it is true that nobody here is LGBT, many folks have LGBT family members and want a space to talk about it.
I don't think programming should be political and push this liberal agenda.	This meeting isn't political; it's about making sure that everyone feels welcome and respected. There are LGBT people in all political parties!
I really hate that this is happening here.	I appreciate your concern, but remember that nobody is forcing anyone to attend the event.

Another strategy is to make use of positive peer pressure. Speak with some of your resident leaders or more active residents and see if you can get them to attend an LGBT event and bring along a friend. Most people don't want to be left out, and if they see their peers engaging in a new and interesting activity, that may be enough to help them get over any initial discomfort.

However it is that your organization decides to respond to questions or pushback from residents, it is important that staff are consistent in their responses and support. A simple response like "We offer a diverse range of activities to meet the needs of our diverse community!" can make sure the resident feels heard, but also makes it clear that the programming is here to stay. As I noted in Box 4.4, one very common response is, "Why would we have this program? Nobody here is gay!" We know that is probably not true, but staff can also respond by noting that many residents may have LGBT family members, and these programs can help them understand their family members' identities and also make those family members feel included in the community.

GOALS AND EVALUATIONS

Setting clear goals and evaluations can also help shape programming. Staff can define these goals as a part of wellness planning or a strategic plan and then create programming with the intention of meeting them. See Box 4.5 for examples.

BOX 4.5   EXAMPLE GOALS AND ACTIVITIES

Goal	Activity
Increase your residents' long-term financial and legal security, as well as advanced planning.	Host a legal clinic with volunteers who are explicitly trained on LGBT cultural competency and legal concerns.

Goal	Activity
Help LGBT residents access preventative care and improve their health.	Engage with community health educators and care managers from a local LGBT center or HIV/AIDS clinic.
Create a sense of community for LGBT residents and an environment where LGBT people are supported if they decide to come out.	Start a GSA or LGBT discussion group.
Attract more potential residents from the LGBT community.	Host a showing of an LGBT movie and invite community members in for a post-movie discussion and food.
Encourage residents to do a letter-writing campaign or volunteer for a cause in the community.	Bring in a panel of non-profit professionals from a variety of causes—such as LGBT rights, racial justice, interfaith movements, or climate activists—to discuss their work and volunteer opportunities.

Many of these ideas can be driven by volunteers or supported by tapping into local resources. Just as new staff are made aware of your community's commitment to LGBT inclusion, new volunteers can be given a similar orientation and can be expected to abide by community standards. Chapter 6 has more information on community standards. You may find resources at your local LGBT community center or group (consider searching through CenterLink, www.lgbtcenters.org), a local HIV/AIDS advocacy group, LGBT chamber of commerce, PFLAG chapter, or college or university LGBT student group. Chapter 14 has other ideas for reaching LGBT board members, and many of those same strategies can be used to attract volunteers and to connect with local supports.

There is no one way to start LGBT programming, so think about your strategic goals and the needs of the residents and start from there. Resident involvement is key, and building off of what is already working is always a good way to start.

SUGGESTIONS

■ Work with the team to decide which approach to programming is the best first step for your community.
■ Let the residents guide programming, and encourage resident leaders to attend the new events.
■ Evaluate programming and meet regularly to assess what is working and what can be changed.
■ Make it clear to residents and staff that attending an LGBT-themed event does not mean that someone is LGBT.

FURTHER READING AND VIEWING

Before You Know It (film) (www.beforeyouknowitfilm.com/).
"GLSEN: Jump Start Your GSA" (www.glsen.org/jumpstart).

"International Gay and Lesbian Travel Association International Pride Calendar" (www.iglta. org/).

"LGBT Programming for Older Adults: A Practical Step-By-Step Guide" (www.lgbtagingcen ter.org/resources/resource.cfm?r=705).

The Trans List (film) (www.hbo.com/documentaries/the-trans-list).

Welcome to Pride: A Practical Guide to Making Pride Parades, Marches and Festivals Age-Friendly (www.sageusa.org/).

REFERENCES

Sahgal, Neha, and Greg Smith. 2009. "A Religious Portrait of African-Americans." *Pew Research Center's Forum on Religion & Public Life.* www.pewforum.org/2009/01/30/a-religious-portrait-of-african-americans/.

LGBT programming and services

5

STAFF OPINIONS, BELIEFS, AND TRAINING

SUMMARY

The staff in most senior living communities come from a wide range of linguistic, cultural, ethnic, political, and religious backgrounds, and each person will have their own opinion about LGBT people and cultures. In order to create a welcoming environment, providers should focus on providing excellent care and services to all residents, including LGBT residents. This may require putting their own beliefs aside, or emphasizing shared beliefs like compassion, empathy, and treating others as they would want to be treated. This chapter outlines the importance of LGBT cultural competency training and how to respond if staff are uncomfortable working with LGBT people.

OBJECTIVES

- Learn why it is important to put your own opinions aside and provide excellent care to all of your residents.
- Examine strategies to identify implicit biases and assumptions and lessen their impact on your work.
- Practice how to balance an employee's right to their own opinions and beliefs with residents' right to fair and equitable treatment.
- Explore options to bring LGBT cultural competency training to your community.

STARTING THE CONVERSATION

Staff are a community's heart and soul. They not only provide care and services to residents, but also set the tone and climate and can develop strong emotional connections with residents and their families. As I noted in the introduction, senior living staff are working in residents' homes, which presents both an opportunity and a responsibility. Creating a welcoming environment for LGBT residents begins with the staff, but many managers and directors worry about how staff will react to efforts to be more inclusive.

If there is one thing I have learned training staff all across the country it's that you can never anticipate who will support LGBT inclusion and who will push back. I am often surprised by how my own assumptions are inaccurate. On one hand, because many people do not openly discuss the topic of diverse sexual orientations and gender identities, it can be hard to know which staff may have LGBT family members or friends, or which may identify as LGBT themselves. On the other hand, you can never anticipate who will be uncomfortable speaking about this topic or have negative feelings about LGBT people. You may have a co-worker who you think will be completely on board with LGBT training, but who surprises you by pushing back and expressing discomfort. That is why the first step toward a more inclusive environment is having open and frank conversations with other staff members and giving them the training they need to work with LGBT older adults.

Be brave! These conversations may feel tense or awkward or they may be welcome and exciting. The only way to find out is to start talking.

GETTING BUY-IN

Who are the people caring for older adults in senior living and other supportive services? Compared to the United States labor force, those working in long-term care are more likely to be women. Of the people working in personal care, nearly 20 percent were born outside of the U.S., and black women comprise one-fourth of this workforce (Argentum 2018). In nursing homes, 80 percent of staff are United States citizens, 13 percent citizens by naturalization, and 7 percent are not citizens. Nationally, direct care staff have a median annual income of just over $21,200 (PHI n.d.). Half of nursing assistants have not completed any education beyond high school, they are three times more likely to be injured on the job than other workers, 17 percent live below the poverty line, and 39 percent make use of some form of public assistance (Campbell 2017). For a deeper dive into the racial and ethnic composition of the long-term care workforce see Bates, Amah, and Coffman 2018.

I mention these statistics because we must remember that many staff are struggling financially while doing a job that is difficult and exhausting. Asking the team to complete additional training may feel like a burden or like they are being asked to do the training because they have done something wrong. It is important that staff are compensated for the time they spend training, supported by supervisors to be off the floor, and told that the purpose of LGBT cultural competency training is to equip them with new and in-demand skills. It is crucial that staff do not think they are being asked to complete this training because they have made a mistake or that it is some kind of punishment. Instead, make it clear that the community is investing in the staff so that they can do their jobs at an even higher level and support them to have the time and space to really pay attention to the training.

BOX 5.1 A CHARGE NURSE'S STORY

When I first heard about the LGBT aging training, I didn't understand why we needed it. We treat everyone equally, no matter who they are. After the training I discussed the topic with my team and I've been surprised at their lack of knowledge about LGBT older people. It has led to some really meaningful and important conversations with my staff, and I'm happy we are all getting some training.

A charge nurse at Wesley Enhanced Living,
Philadelphia PA

CHOOSING A TRAINING PROVIDER OR CONSULTANT

LGBT cultural competency trainings often touch on terminology, the history of LGBT experience, case studies or testimonials, information on legal protections, and best practices. Longer or more sophisticated trainings may also include information on how to respond if you see another staffer or vendor acting in a negative or biased way (Meyer 2011). Some providers prefer in-person sessions, others on-demand, and more and more training organizations are offering on-demand interactive trainings. I have found it works best when communities integrate LGBT training into their existing training processes and patterns, using whatever formats or learning management systems the staff are accustomed to for their other professional training.

You may have staff with some LGBT experience and expertise, but it can be helpful to bring in outside trainers and consultants. An outside consultant will have experience across a variety of senior living settings and provide a level of external authority that an internal staff person may not carry. There are a number of organizations that offer LGBT aging cultural competency training, including

■ SAGECare;
■ The LGBT Aging Project;
■ Project Visibility;
■ Generations Aging with Pride;
■ Transgender Aging Network;
■ Training to Serve;
■ Eldersource;
■ Openhouse.

And many local LGBT community centers, advocacy groups, or health and human service providers also have LGBT cultural competency training—some designed specifically for aging service providers.

When deciding on a training program it is important that you assess their expertise, ensuring that they are well versed not only in the needs of gay and lesbian older adults, but also bisexual and transgender residents. Several training programs have been shown to have statistically significant positive changes in staff beliefs, knowledge, and attitudes toward LGBT older adults (Porter and Krinsky 2014; Leyva, Breshears, and Ringstad 2014; Doherty et al. 2016), and a robust evaluation program with proven results is another good way to assess a potential training program. Always ask for evaluation information, testimonials, feedback from participants, and examples of how the training has made a positive difference for other organizations.

BOX 5.2   HOW LGBT INCLUSION CAN CONNECT YOU TO THE WIDER COMMUNITY

Aldersgate is continuing care retirement community located in Charlotte, North Carolina. Our community is in a part of the city distinguished by a population that is diverse in terms of socioeconomic status, race, religion, sexual orientation, gender identity, and country of origin—all of which make East Charlotte beautiful and Aldersgate unique. As an organization we spend each and every day working on how we can continue to live by our mission of honoring elders.

In 2018 we earned our SAGECare Platinum credential. The SAGECare workshop was mandatory for all Aldersgate teammates and contractors. We had our leadership and all of our director- and manager-level staff attend the in-person, four-hour trainings provided by SAGE. The rest of our staff completed a 90-minute workshop that I taught almost 50 times to make sure we reached all of our staff. We hosted informational sessions for residents about the SAGE training and about our work as an organization to be a place where all of our current and future residents can be who they are. The sessions were well attended and welcomed by many of our residents. We also discussed the training at our semi-monthly coffee with the chief executive officer and chief diversity and inclusion officer. We knew it was important to have buy-in from the residents and for them to see this commitment coming from the top.

After training, we started to intentionally partner with LGBTQ local and national organizations. Those organizations include HRC, Charlotte Pride, PFLAG, RAIN, EqualityNC, and many more. We were the first retirement community to have ever participated in the Charlotte Pride Parade and Pride Weekend. We've seen an increase in the number of LGBTQ residents, and our staff and residents are excited that Aldersgate is becoming known for being open and inclusive. The work that we have been doing in the past year has not gone unnoticed. Our efforts to build a welcoming LGBTQ community and our partnering with SAGE have increased our potential residents list, tours, and depositors by about 10 percent. The LGBTQ consumer impact is being felt each and every day at Aldersgate and in our wonderful east Charlotte.

Veronica Calderon
Chief Diversity & Inclusion Officer
Aldersgate: Charlotte, NC

EXPLICIT AND IMPLICIT BIAS

Learning facts, terms, history, and best practices are important aspects of a training program, but another less tangible goal is to make staff more aware of their own personal biases and how they impact care.

Bias is when a person has a preference for or prejudice against another person or group of people, typically in a way that is unfair. Explicit bias is when the person with a prejudice knows that they are acting in a biased manner. For example, if a straight resident explicitly refuses to share a dining room table with a gay resident, the straight resident is acting out of explicit bias. Implicit bias operates at the unconscious level, meaning we often do not realize we are acting in a biased way (Devine 1989). For example, one negative and inaccurate idea about people living with HIV is that they are more sexually active than other people or that they may make people around them sick. A person who has internalized this negative bias might feel vaguely uneasy around someone who they know is HIV positive and keep their distance or avoid physical contact, likely without realizing why they are doing so.

Another way to think about this is in terms of stereotypes. Sometimes we recognize when we are thinking according to a stereotype. Other times, that stereotype influences our actions without us knowing it. Stereotypes are often negative, but stereotypes that might be seen as positive, such as the "model minority myth" (the idea that certain minority groups, for example Asian-Americans, are particularly successful), can be harmful because they oversimplify diverse communities. That is to say, whether our stereotypes are positive or negative, if we treat people as stereotypes we are not seeing them as unique individuals.

We all have different biases—each and every one of us. We make thousands of small and quick decisions every day, and it is impossible to grow into adulthood without internalizing negative and inaccurate biases of some kind. Research shows that there are ways to reduce the impact of implicit bias, often by helping people see their biases and understand how they are impacting others (Devine et al. 2012). There are also researchers who question our ability to measure and address these biases or whether changes in implicit bias have any impact on behavior, so this is not a settled area of research (Bartlett 2017). That said, I think the distinction between explicit and implicit bias is helpful when training people to be more inclusive. No training or activity can eliminate our biases, but they can help create an environment where people can point out and address one another's biases in respectful and constructive ways.

These implicit biases can also lead us to make assumptions. For example, Jane is chatting with a new resident, Alisha, who lives alone in the community. Alisha mentions having grandchildren, and in a follow-up question Jane asks, "What was your husband's name?" Jane's question reflects an implicit bias or stereotype that all grandmothers are heterosexual, or that if you are a grandmother you were probably at one point married to a man. This may be the case for many grandmothers, but in fact Alisa is a lesbian and raised her children with her female partner. Now Alisha is in the position of needing to correct Jane, and she may decide it is not worth the trouble or be unsure how Jane will react. LGBT cultural competency training can give Jane a wider perspective on identities and relationships, so instead of assuming Alisha was married to a man, she might simply ask, "Tell me more about your family and community," which will make it easier for Alisha to be open about herself. After being trained, if Jane hears other staff asking questions that reflect bias or assumptions, she can point that out to them and suggest other ways to ask questions.

PUSHBACK FROM STAFF

As I said previously, you can never guess which of the staff may push back against LGBT inclusion. One clear pattern I see is managers making assumptions about staff's openness based on the staff person's racial, ethnic, or religious identity or where they are from. Many front-line care providers are immigrants to the United States and may be moving from places with negative cultural views of LGBT people or places where same-sex sexual contact is illegal, or they may have deeply rooted religious views against LGBT identities. Of course, that will not be true for many immigrants, and there are plenty of communities and organized religions in the United States that are still hostile to LGBT people. It is important not to make assumptions about how your staff will react based on where they are from or their religion. We all have different biases, and it is impossible to predict a person's reaction to LGBT training and inclusion based on their country of origin, religion, or any other characteristic.

Staff may react poorly to efforts like training, LGBT programming, inclusive imagery, or nondiscrimination policies for several reasons. They could be expressing a religious or political conviction, they may have personal discomfort with LGBT people, they may not understand the importance of the training and resent being taken off the floor, or they may simply be overworked and feel overburdened. If staff are being vocal and pushing back against training the first step is to determine what is behind the pushback. Is it a deeply held conviction, or are they complaining to blow off steam? One-on-one conversations can help managers get to the bottom of the complaints and craft a response.

BOX 5.3   STAFF WHO REFUSE TO PROVIDE SERVICES TO LGBT RESIDENTS

What can you do if a staff person flat-out refuses to provide services to an LGBT resident? First, determine if there is any abuse or unequitable treatment happening in the community. Treating any resident poorly or providing them with unequitable or substandard care is elder abuse and should be met with the appropriate response to end the abuse.

If there is no abuse, but the staff person refuses to care for a specific resident, there are a number of things to consider and questions to ask:

- Always center the rights and needs of the LGBT elder.
- Treat the situation in the same way you would if a staff person refused to work with a resident because of a disability or dementia diagnosis, race, ethnicity, or religion.

- ■ Determine if this is a firm conviction or a personality conflict. What is the root of the request? Is it really because the resident is LGBT, is there a personality clash, or is something else going on?
- ■ Is there the possibility for reassignment, and what does the resident want?
- ■ Is this person's request incompatible with your mission to treat all residents with respect, and if so is it grounds for disciplinary action or separation from the organization?

Staff have a right to feel comfortable in the workplace, but that can never overshadow your community's commitment to providing equitable care for all residents. Consider looking at your existing policies and practices to make sure that they are inclusive of LGBT residents and that staff are aware of their responsibility to provide care to all residents.

The two most common forms of pushback I have heard in the field are

"I don't understand why these people need special treatment."

and

"I don't see why we need this training; I treat everyone the same and it doesn't matter to me if they are LGBT."

As we discussed in Chapter 1, both of these comments confuse equality with equity. If the goal of inclusion was to treat everyone the same, then it might appear to be special treatment to devote additional resources to LGBT training and outreach. However, when we remember that LGBT people face unique barriers to accessing services, as well as unique fears about being open, we can see that providing LGBT older adults with equitable care and services does require this extra effort. Many providers are not familiar with LGBT people or communities. Without training they may think they are treating residents the same when in fact they are making assumptions that create a negative environment for LGBT residents.

If the source of the pushback is a staff person's religion, while we should all respect one another's religious convictions, it must be emphasized that religion cannot be used to justify or validate unequitable or substandard treatment of any resident. I have seen managers, especially if they are working within an organization that has a religious identity, effectively articulate their support for LGBT inclusion using religious language and concepts. That said, in the majority of cases I have found that trying to convince people using religious or political arguments is ineffective and can deepen existing tensions between staff. That is why I focus on professional ethical standards to anchor the importance of caring for all people, and the skill of putting aside one's beliefs or judgements, instead emphasizing that we all deserve to be treated with respect. I usually say something like, "This training is not political and my goal is not to change your beliefs. My goal is to give you specialized skills that you need to reach a vulnerable population and do your job at the highest level." These are also opportunities for people to practice empathy. Working with an LGBT resident may seem new to some staff, but they will quickly see that the new resident is a person who also has needs, fears, joys, and hopes and that we have more in common than we might think. Emphasizing that we are working in these people's home and have a responsibility to help residents feel supported and at home are important ways to build strong, caring relationships.

Keeping the focus on professional development and reaching vulnerable older adults can help re-center our commitment to care work. Remember that many of your fellow staff do this work because they are caring people focused on helping others.

SUGGESTIONS

■ Spend time noticing patterns in your behavior or actions that may reflect an implicit bias. Consider how your beliefs and opinions may contribute to the way you care for your residents.

■ Learn about LGBT communities and familiarize yourself with the LGBT experience; see if there are similarities with your own experience. This can help build a reservoir of connection and empathy.

■ Incorporate routine LGBT cultural competency training into new staff orientation and annual training programs.

■ Meet with staff to discuss your community's commitment to LGBT inclusion and create a space to hear any questions or concerns.

FURTHER READING AND VIEWING

Biased: Uncovering the Hidden Prejudice that Shapes What We See, Think, and Do by Jennifer L. Eberhardt.

"Building Respect for LGBT Older Adults" (www.lgbtagingcenter.org/).

Hinrichs, Kate L.M., and Tammi Vacha-Haase. 2010. "Staff Perceptions of Same-Gender Sexual Contacts in Long-Term Care Facilities." *Journal of Homosexuality* 57 (6): 776–89. https://doi.org/10.1080/00918369.2010.485877.

"Learning to Address Implicit Bias Towards LGBTQ Patients: Case Scenarios" (www.lgbthealtheducation.org/).

"National LGBT Health Education Center" (www.lgbthealtheducation.org/).

"Project Implicit—Harvard Implicit Bias Tests" (https://implicit.harvard.edu/).

REFERENCES

Argentum. 2018. "The Senior Living Employee: A Socioeconomic Portrait of Today's Worker." Alexandria, VA: Argentum. www.argentum.org/wp-content/uploads/2018/05/Senior-Living-Resident-Profile-WhitePaper.pdf.

Bartlett, Tom. 2017. "Can We Really Measure Implicit Bias? Maybe Not—The Chronicle of Higher Education." *The Chronicle of Higher Education*. January 5, 2017. www.chronicle.com/article/Can-We-Really-Measure-Implicit/238807.

Bates, Timothy, Ginachukwu Amah, and Janet Coffman. 2018. "Racial/Ethnic Diversity in the Long-Term Care Workforce." San Francisco: Health Workforce Research Center on Long-Term Care, University of California San Francisco. https://healthworkforce.ucsf.edu/sites/healthworkforce.ucsf.edu/files/REPORT-2018.HWRC_diversity_.4-18.pdf.

Campbell, Stephen. 2017. "U.S. Nursing Assistants Employed in Nursing Homes: Key Facts." *PHI (Paraprofessional Healthcare Institute)*. https://phinational.org/resource/u-s-nursing-assistants-employed-in-nursing-homes-key-facts/.

Devine, Patricia G. 1989. "Stereotypes and Prejudice: Their Automatic and Controlled Components." *Journal of Personality and Social Psychology* 56 (1): 5–18. https://doi.org/10.1037/0022-3514.56.1.5.

Devine, Patricia G., Patrick S. Forscher, Anthony J. Austin, and William T.L. Cox. 2012. "Long-Term Reduction in Implicit Race Bias: A Prejudice Habit-Breaking Intervention." *Journal of Experimental Social Psychology* 48 (6): 1267–78. https://doi.org/10.1016/j.jesp.2012.06.003.

Doherty, Meredith, Tim R. Johnston, Hilary Meyer, and Nancy Giunta. 2016. "SAGE's National Resource Center on LGBT Aging Is Training a Culturally Competent Aging Network." *Generations* 40 (2): 78–9.

Leyva, Valerie L., Elizabeth M. Breshears, and Robin Ringstad. 2014. "Assessing the Efficacy of LGBT Cultural Competency Training for Aging Services Providers in California's Central Valley." *Journal of Gerontological Social Work* 57 (2–4): 335–48. https://doi.org/10.1080/01634372.2013.872215.

Meyer, H. 2011. "Safe Spaces? The Need for LGBT Cultural Competency in Aging Services." *Public Policy & Aging Report* 21 (3): 24–7. https://doi.org/10.1093/ppar/21.3.24.

PHI. n.d. "Workforce Data Center." *PHI* (blog). Accessed August 9, 2018. https://phinational.org/policy-research/workforce-data-center/.

Porter, Kristen E., and Lisa Krinsky. 2014. "Do LGBT Aging Trainings Effectuate Positive Change in Mainstream Elder Service Providers?" *Journal of Homosexuality* 61 (1): 197–216. https://doi.org/10.1080/00918369.2013.835618.

6

ADDRESSING BULLYING AND CONFLICT BETWEEN RESIDENTS

SUMMARY

Many people living in your community, as well as some staff, came of age during a time when being LGBT was taboo or considered a mental illness, and they may still hold negative views about LGBT people. LGBT community members may be more vulnerable to bullying or other forms of aggression and discrimination by their neighbors. This chapter outlines ways to identify, prevent, and respond to conflict between residents and how to support staff in creating an environment where everyone can live free from bullying.

OBJECTIVES

- Learn the definition of bullying and how to distinguish between conflict and bullying.
- Consider preventative policies and practices to help stop bullying before it starts.
- Learn several techniques for addressing conflict or systemic bullying.

ANY AND ALL COMMUNITIES WILL HAVE SOME CONFLICT

Former United States Surgeon General Vivek Murthy says that loneliness is now an epidemic (McGregor 2017), and in one survey nearly half of Americans reported feeling lonely or left out some or all of the time (CIGNA 2018). Isolation and loneliness can have a negative impact on a person's physical and mental health (Singer 2018; Klinenberg 2016; Tanskanen and Anttila 2016), and LGBT older adults are more likely to be isolated than their non-LGBT peers (Choi and Meyer 2016). Moving into a senior living community is a great opportunity to reduce isolation by creating pleasant, comfortable, and engaging places where people have the opportunity to socialize and form strong relationships.

Living in a community also involves different personalities, perspectives, and preferences—all of which can lead to conflict. It is unusual to live and socialize with the same group of people all day every day, and this makes senior living a unique environment where nerves may get frayed and conflict can spark quickly.

Minor conflicts like bickering and complaining are a normal part of community living, but this chapter looks at how to respond when everyday conflict rises to the level of bullying. There is not much research on bullying between older people, but studies suggest that approximately 20 percent of residents in senior living experience bullying, and we do know that many LGBT older adults fear bullying and abuse from staff and other residents (Bonifas 2016b; Trompetter, Scholte, and Westerhof 2011; Fredriksen-Goldsen 2011; Houghton 2018). As I travel the country conducting trainings I often hear managers say, "I'm not worried about how my staff will respond to an LGBT person moving into our community—I'm worried about how the other residents will react!" This is a very real concern, so what tools do staff need to help make sure that all residents, including LGBT residents, are not being bullied?

WHAT IS THE DIFFERENCE BETWEEN CONFLICT AND BULLYING?

Dan Olweus (1993) and many other researchers and advocates agree that bullying is defined by three criteria:

1. The bully is intentionally harming the target. The harm may be physical (pinching, hitting, slapping, intimidation), verbal (name-calling, yelling, insulting), or social (gossiping, spreading rumors, isolating or shunning).
2. The harm is committed by a person who has more power than the target. This power may be physical strength, social status, better health, more money, or anything else that gives the bully an advantage over the target.
3. There is the threat of continued or repeated harm. The harm is not a one-time event.

This three-part definition can help distinguish bullying from other behavior. If a frustrated resident makes a hurtful remark, that is not necessarily bullying because it may not happen again. A person with dementia may become physically aggressive, but that attack is not on purpose or targeting a specific person, and many people with dementia cannot remember their behavior so it is not part of an intentional pattern.

This definition also shows us that some behavior that staff may usually ignore can be considered bullying. If a group of three women always stop another woman from joining them at a table for dinner, that is repeated and intentional social isolation. A staff person may initially tell the woman to just ignore the three women and find another table, but this repeated exclusion could be part of a larger pattern of bullying. Accidently using the wrong name or pronoun when speaking to a transgender resident is not necessarily bullying, but intentionally doing so is an example of verbal bullying.

Training staff on this definition will help them distinguish between one-time hurts or conflict between equals and bullying behavior. Moreover, teaching this definition to residents will help them see if they are being bullied. Someone who is being bullied may think that the hurtful behavior is unpleasant but simply "how things are" or a "part of life" and all they can do is "toughen up" and get through it. People who are also minorities may have internalized negative messages or stigmas about their identity, for example, coming to believe negative stereotypes about themselves or feeling worn down by the discrimination they have faced over their lifetime. This can make people more likely to accept the abuse rather than stand up for themselves. Low self-esteem, fear of reprisals, and lack of support are also reasons that people do not report bullying. Understanding what bullying looks like and naming it can empower residents to stand up for their right to not be bullied.

BOX 6.1 BULLYING CASE STUDY

Scenario

Estelle is one of your residents. She recently transitioned into using a wheelchair to travel between her room and the dining room. Whenever she goes down the hallway she whizzes past Joan and Maria, a married couple who recently moved into your community, yelling, "Out of my way, ladies!"

Estelle only does this to Joan and Maria. This is alarming to the two women, one of whom walks very slowly. Other residents tend to laugh at Estelle's performance, but you notice the two women are growing increasingly perturbed, and they have started arriving to lunch early to avoid Estelle.

Is this bullying?

Let's take a look at the three components of bullying:

1. Does Estelle have more power than Joan and Maria?

   Estelle has lived in the community longer, and she might have more social power because Joan and Maria are new and may be a little isolated because they are a same-sex couple. The fact that most people condone Estelle's behavior, while not recognizing its negative impact on the couple, also implies that she has more social power.

2. Is the harm intentional?

   Yes, it is clear that Estelle is doing this on purpose only to Joan and Maria.

3. Is the harm being repeated?

   Yes, this is becoming routine and beginning to force Joan and Maria to change their behaviors.

What could be causing the bullying?

Estelle may be lashing out because of her recent transition to using a wheelchair. Zooming down the hallway and seeing Joan and Maria move out of her way can make her feel like she has some control or power, even though she can no longer walk to the dining room herself. It could also be the case that she does not like the two women because they are in a same-sex relationship, and this is how she is making that feeling known.

How can staff respond?

Make sure Estelle knows she is having a negative impact on the women and that she cannot move down the hallway at a speed that is dangerous for others. Check in with Joan and Maria to let them know staff are addressing the behavior. Finally, sit down with Estelle to try to get to the bottom of the behavior and address the root causes.

WHY DO PEOPLE BULLY, AND HOW DO THEY PICK THEIR TARGETS?

There is no single reason why someone becomes a bully. Some bullies were themselves bullied and learned the behavior through that experience. Some people bully to gain a benefit, such as increased social power, attention from staff, access to activities or services, or special treatment. Others bully because they are biased and want to cause harm to a person they do not like, for example, bullying an LGBT person to make them leave the room.

A resident may also become a bully to gain or maintain a sense of control and power within the community. If a new resident used to be a successful business executive she may be feeling insecure, vulnerable, or even powerless in her new environment, and bullying is a way to regain a sense of control and agency. Other factors that contribute to bullying behavior include

- A change in environment, such as moving from home to a community setting;
- Retirement or other changes to identity or social role;

- Significant loss, such as the death of a spouse or other loved one;
- Reaction to ageism and feeling invisible or less valuable;
- Changes in health or mobility, including cognitive decline or needing to use a cane, walker, wheelchair, or hearing aids.

Bullying behavior may have an underlying cause such as depression, anxiety, chronic pain, or the beginning stages of memory loss, and the negative behavior may be a way to compensate for or hide these unaddressed issues (Bonifas 2016a).

There is also no one characteristic that defines the targets of bullying. A resident may be targeted because they are different from the majority of other residents, because they are seen to be weak, because they are new, or simply because the bully does not like them. The fact that bullying is repeated behavior means that targets often become fearful, withdraw, change their behavior to avoid the bully, or become isolated, depressive, hypervigilant, or anxious. Left unaddressed, bullying can negatively impact the climate of a community, creating a negative and fearful atmosphere, lowering resident satisfaction and employee morale.

BULLYING VERSUS ABUSE

In addition to distinguishing between bullying and conflict, it is important to note a third, related behavior: abuse. Elder abuse can take the form of bullying, and both might involve physical harm or harassment. The key difference is that elder abuse involves an older adult who is somehow dependent on the abuser, whereas with bullying both the bully and target may be older adults with vulnerabilities and dependencies, but the target is not dependent on the bully. Chapter 13 goes into more detail on the various legal protections that apply specifically to LGBT residents, but all older adults have the right to be free from abuse and the right to be treated with respect. State and federal laws criminalize elder abuse, and some states are including bullying in their definition of elder abuse. Even if your state does not define bullying as a form of elder abuse, both merit immediate response, and residents have the right to be free from both abuse and bullying.

BOX 6.2   BULLYING CASE STUDY

After his long-term partner, Tim, died suddenly of a heart attack, George moved into a suburban Boston assisted living facility. Tim had cared for George over the last few years after a cancer diagnosis led to surgery and ongoing medical issues. George, a retired high school teacher, was struggling to adapt to his new living situation, as well as the loss of his partner.

A care assistant overheard another resident, John, say to several other residents within George's hearing that he didn't want to be seated near George in the dining room as he was a "queer and might carry disease."

The assistant was uncertain as to what to say or do, so spoke to the nursing supervisor. When questioned by the supervisor, other staff reported they had heard John make similar comments previously. The nursing supervisor brought the staff together to train them on how to respond to comments that smacked of bullying or harassment, whether directed at George or others.

Staff were instructed to say, "In this community we don't speak about people in that way. We welcome people from diverse backgrounds and sexual orientations and statements like John's violated the code of behavior that all residents signed on admission." It is important that staff be polite, but clear in their messaging and that it was imparted in front of the other residents and that the targeted individual heard it, as well.

Practitioners have learned the importance of having a clear code of behavior that spells out inappropriate language/actions, including bullying, and that all staff be empowered and trained in an appropriate response. Being called out in front of bystanders weakens the power of the bully and provides needed support to the person being targeted.

Following staff's intervention, the next time they overheard John make a disparaging, homophobic comment, several residents reached out to support George, with one asking his advice about how to respond to his teenage grandson who had just told him that he was gay. Gradually George found a group of residents that he enjoyed spending time with and became a leader of the resident council.

Marsha Frankel, LICSW
Consultant, Psychotherapist, Trainer
Former Clinical Director of Senior Services at Jewish Family & Children's Service

HOW TO RESPOND TO BULLYING

Every bully is unique, and responses must be tailored to the people involved. The following are some general recommendations; they are not exhaustive. For additional recommendations, including how to conduct a bullying questionnaire, as well as a more in-depth discussion of these recommendations see Robin Bonifas's book *Bullying among Older Adults: How to Recognize and Address an Unseen Epidemic*, specifically Chapters 4 and 5.

Responding in the moment

The first things to do are stop the bullying, make it clear to everyone that the behavior is unacceptable, and de-escalate the situation. If the bullying is physical or verbal someone may need to separate the people involved. If the bullying is social, staff can check in with the person being harmed to see if they are OK, help the target find a new activity, or escort them into a different space. Regular training for all staff and volunteers is important to make sure that everyone, not only management, has the skills needed to stop and de-escalate bullying when they see it.

Following up

After the incident follow up with everyone involved individually and privately. When speaking with the bully, try to keep the focus on the impact of the bully's behavior, rather than on the bully themselves. The goal is to make sure that they understand their actions are causing harm. For example, if you hear a resident make a homophobic comment, rather than responding with "That was homophobic" or "Stop saying bigoted things," you could say, "That is a hurtful word, and when you use language like that it makes others feel uncomfortable." Keeping the focus on the bully's impact on the community, rather than judging the bully as a person, can help keep the bully from becoming angry or defensive, while inviting them to develop empathy for the target of their hurtful behavior.

These conversations are also an opportunity to see if there is an underlying cause to the hurtful behavior. If a bully targets people using walkers, the bully may have unaddressed anxieties about their own mobility and aging, and addressing those fears can be the first step toward building empathy.

When speaking with the target, reinforce that what happened is not acceptable and that staff are working to address the situation. Stay in touch, check back, and communicate any changes or actions staff are taking to prevent future harms. Follow-through is essential to making sure residents know that staff take bullying seriously. Residents may not report bullying because they are afraid the bully will "get even" and intensify the harm. Consistent follow-up from staff demonstrates to everyone that staff are aware of the risk of reprisal and any future bullying will not be tolerated.

Finally, consider speaking with bystanders or holding a town-hall or open discussion on the topic of bullying. Most people, including bullies, have been the targets of bullying at some point in their lives. Asking residents to reflect on their experience and the kind of community they want to live in can increase empathy and empower bystanders and targets to stand up in the future.

Policies

Creating a strong culture against bullying begins with a code of conduct that outlines community standards and a gradual disciplinary structure if people are bullying or otherwise causing harm. This statement should include your community's nondiscrimination policy that explicitly mentions sexual orientation, gender identity, and gender expression as protected categories, or include explicit mention of the rights of minority groups including LGBT people. Staff and volunteers should also agree to these codes.

BOX 6.3   SAMPLE LGBT-INCLUSIVE CODE OF CONDUCT

SAGE operates several LGBT senior centers across New York City. The following is part of the SAGE Centers—Code of conduct rules document. All new participants read and sign this document. This is important because it sets consistent expectations, and when participants violate these norms staff can use this document as a part of follow-up conversations. Note that it mentions LGBT people, lists specific expectations around names, pronouns, and LGBT identities, and outlines the steps staff will take when they see hurtful behavior.

SAGE Centers—Code of conduct rules

SAGE Centers provide a safe, warm and welcoming space for LGBT people and allies, age 60 and older. The SAGE Centers were created to foster an environment for constituents to participate, socialize, learn, and volunteer. To ensure the comfort and safety of the community, the following applies to participants, staff, consultants, volunteers and guests who attend any SAGE programming.

1. SAGE supports an individual's right to express their chosen identity and experience. This includes respecting and using an individual's chosen name, pronoun (e.g. he, she, they, etc.) and identities (e.g. lesbian, gay, bisexual, asexual, transgender, queer, etc.). Behavior or language that infringes upon this right is prohibited.
2. Behavior, presentation, and actions which create an unsafe environment (e.g., not responding to direction by staff, verbally or physically aggressive behavior) are not allowed. This includes communication on SAGE social media platforms, as per SAGE policy.
3. Actions, behavior, and language that is or may be construed as abusive, threatening, harassing and/or insulting is not allowed.

Corrective action for violation of SAGE code of conduct rules

1st Incident—Verbal Warning: SAGE staff or designee will address the situation and issue a verbal warning, as necessary. The incident will be documented in SAGE files and a copy will be made available.

2nd Incident—Written Warning: Site manager or their designee will address the situation and issue a written warning, as necessary. The incident will be documented and a copy will be provided.

3rd Incident—Suspension: Site manager or their designee will address the situation and issue a suspension in writing, as necessary. Time period of suspension is determined on a case by case basis. The incident will be documented and a copy will be provided to participant.

Consider creating an anonymous way for residents and staff to report bullying. Targets of bullying may be afraid that if they come forward the bullying will get worse. LGBT people may be experiencing anti-LGBT bullying but not want to tell staff if they do not want to come out as LGBT or discuss their LGBT identity. A bully may also be harming the target by threatening to out them to the rest of the community. A comment box, online form, or other anonymous reporting option can help staff keep track of bullying behavior without making the target feel vulnerable to retaliation. Training all staff on all shifts is also important to make sure that bullying behavior is not happening when management is not around.

IT'S A BALANCING ACT

It can be challenging to know when to intervene and when to let people sort out their own conflict. Some staff may not take action because they do not want to make a bigger deal out of something that is normal conflict, or blow a small fight out of proportion. Staff may also be worried about forcing people to do things that they do not want to do or forcing them to share the same space. For example, people often ask, "If someone doesn't want to eat dinner at the same table as a same-sex couple, isn't that their right?" We do all have the right to decide who we spend time with, and to avoid people we do not like. This same-sex couple may also have zero desire to share a table with a person who is uncomfortable with them. This is where the definition of bullying is helpful. If all people involved simply want to avoid one another, they probably have the same amount of power. If, however, a clique forms and the same-sex couple can never find a place to sit, or if they are feeling marginalized in the community, then the conflict has become bullying and needs to be addressed.

Each bully is unique. By identifying and discussing bullying behavior staff can work to prevent it from happening, and they can rehabilitate the bully to direct their energy into healthier and safer activities. Like much disruptive behavior, bullying is the expression of a need, and with patience and care staff can help the resident satisfy that need without harming other residents or the larger community.

SUGGESTIONS

- Conflict, bullying, or other harm should be addressed in the moment and then by following up with each person individually and privately, focusing on the impact of the event rather than the people involved.
- Have resident and employee guidelines outlining clear expectations related to LGBT inclusion, bullying, and corrective action.
- Always report any conflict, bullying, or harm to a supervisor.

FURTHER READING AND VIEWING

Bullying among Older Adults: How to Recognize and Address an Unseen Epidemic by Robin P. Bonifas.

"Bullying among Seniors (and Not the High School Kind): A Prevention and Surveillance Resource for Assisted Living Providers" (www.ahcancal.org/).

Microaggressions in Everyday Life: Race, Gender, and Sexual Orientation by Derald Wing Sue.

"Residents' Rights and the LGBT Community: Know YOUR Rights as a Nursing Home Resident" (http://ltcombudsman.org/uploads/files/support/lgbt-residents-rights-fact-sheet.pdf).

REFERENCES

Bonifas, Robin P. 2016a. *Bullying among Older Adults: How to Recognize and Address an Unseen Epidemic*. Baltimore, MD: Health Professions Press, Inc.

———. 2016b. "The Prevalence of Elder Bullying and Impact on LGBT Elders." In *Handbook of LGBT Elders*, edited by Debra A. Harley and Pamela B. Teaster, 359–72. Cham: Springer International Publishing. https://doi.org/10.1007/978-3-319-03623-6.

Choi, Soon Kyu, and Ilan H. Meyer. 2016. "LGBT Aging: A Review of Research Findings, Needs, and Policy Implications." *The Williams Institute: UCLA School of Law*. https://williamsinstitute.law.ucla.edu/wp-content/uploads/LGBT-Aging-A-Review.pdf.

CIGNA. 2018. "CIGNA U.S. Loneliness Index: Survey of 20,000 Americans Examining Behaviors Driving Loneliness in the United States." *CIGNA*. www.multivu.com/players/English/8294451-cigna-us-loneliness-survey/docs/IndexReport_1524069371598-173525450.pdf.

Fredriksen-Goldsen, K.I. 2011. "Resilience and Disparities among Lesbian, Gay, Bisexual, and Transgender Older Adults." *Public Policy & Aging Report* 21 (3): 3–7. https://doi.org/10.1093/ppar/21.3.3.

Houghton, Angela. 2018. "Maintaining Dignity: A Survey of LGBT Adults Age 45 and Older." *AARP Research* (March). https://doi.org/10.26419/res.00217.001.

Klinenberg, Eric. 2016. "Social Isolation, Loneliness, and Living Alone: Identifying the Risks for Public Health." *American Journal of Public Health* 106 (5): 786–87. https://doi.org/10.2105/AJPH.2016.303166.

McGregor, Jena. 2017. "This Former Surgeon General Says There's a 'Loneliness Epidemic' and Work Is Partly to Blame." *Washington Post*. October 4, 2017. www.washingtonpost.com/news/on-leadership/wp/2017/10/04/this-former-surgeon-general-says-theres-a-loneliness-epidemic-and-work-is-partly-to-blame/.

Olweus, Dan. 1993. *Bullying at School: What We Know and What We Can Do*. Oxford, UK; Cambridge, MA: Blackwell.

Singer, Clifford. 2018. "Health Effects of Social Isolation and Loneliness." *Journal of Aging Life Care* (spring). www.aginglifecarejournal.org/health-effects-of-social-isolation-and-loneliness/.

Tanskanen, Jussi, and Timo Anttila. 2016. "A Prospective Study of Social Isolation, Loneliness, and Mortality in Finland." *American Journal of Public Health* 106 (11): 2042–48. https://doi.org/10.2105/AJPH.2016.303431.

Trompetter, Hester, Ron Scholte, and Gerben Westerhof. 2011. "Resident-to-Resident Relational Aggression and Subjective Well-Being in Assisted Living Facilities." *Aging & Mental Health* 15 (1): 59–67. https://doi.org/10.1080/13607863.2010.501059.

NAVIGATING FAMILY DYNAMICS

7

SUMMARY

Many LGBT older adults come out later in life, often after having been married and having children. If they come out of the closet these LGBT older adults may have strained relationships with their families of origin, and often rely on chosen family or families of choice for their care and companionship. Additionally, they may be in long-term partnerships but not have any legal protection, such as marriage or power of attorney. This chapter orients staff to LGBT family structures and care networks, while also preparing staff to handle potential conflicts between residents and their families of origin.

OBJECTIVES

- Understand LGBT care networks and family structures outside of the typical nuclear family.
- Consider how to center the rights and interests of the resident, even when their family of origin is hostile or has competing interests.
- Consider why many LGBT older adults wait until later in life to come out of the closet.
- Learn how to keep residents connected to their chosen family and friends.

"WE ARE FAMILY. I'VE GOT ALL MY SISTERS WITH ME!"

Families come in all shapes and sizes, and while many people still think of a husband, wife, and children when they hear the word "family," our society is slowly embracing different definitions of what it means to be a family.

Family members play an important role in a resident's wellbeing. From moving in to visiting to overseeing their loved one's care, families are often very present in a community and can help provide useful information to care providers and give the resident a sense of continuity and connection to their broader community. Too narrow a definition of family will make it difficult for staff to ensure that a resident is surrounded by their real support network. This is important not only for LGBT residents, but also for other residents who may also have support structures that are different than the nuclear family.

BOX 7.1 JANET AND GORDON FORBES' STORY

The diversity group in our community put on an event where the parents of LGBT children were asked to tell their stories and talk about what it is like to have a child come out. Our son is gay and he visits us regularly. He's a musician and everyone loves it when he gives us a mini-concert.

When the committee first approached us to be speakers, we were a little nervous, and as the day came closer we actually thought it was going to be really boring. Well, were we ever wrong! We were overwhelmed by the response and interest, lots of people asked questions, and after the event a number of couples approached us, including several couples known to be conservative, to share with us privately that they also have an LGBT child.

You need to start the conversation! You never know who has an LGBT family member, and it's only through dialogue that we can come together in our shared experiences.

Janet and Gordon Forbes

When discussing the experiences of LGBT people, we often make a distinction between a person's family of origin and their chosen family or family of choice. A person's family of origin is their biological or legal family members: mother, father, siblings, cousins, adoptive parents, etc. Nobody can choose their parents or the members of their family of origin. Importantly, unless the resident is married or has a power of attorney, these are the people who have automatic decision-making authority in the event that a resident is incapacitated, and they will often inherit property and be able to make decisions about a resident's possessions, assets, medical care, and memorial or funeral services.

By contrast, a chosen family is a group of people who are probably not legally or biologically related to the resident but who are, for all intents and purposes, their family—their closest supports. A classic example is the television show *The Golden Girls*. Only Sofia and Dorothy are biologically related, but together with Blanche and Rose all four women live as a family and bicker, fight, laugh, and support one another like any other family.

This distinction between family of origin and chosen family is essential because many LGBT people have very strained relationships, or no relationships at all, with their family of origin. Coming out is difficult at any age, and being older does not protect you from family rejection. It is common to hear of people who come out later in life, often after a divorce, the death of a spouse, retirement, or after their children have left home. A partner or parent's new identity is often a shock to their family of origin, and hurt feelings or anti-LGBT opinions may lead to distanced relationships. LGBT older adults may choose to come out, they may be outed by another person, or if they are living with dementia they may begin to act on same-sex desires or express their gender in a new way but not be able to understand that they are coming out or surprising their family. Many LGBT older adults experienced family rejection when they came out and may have never repaired those bonds. This means that they may prefer to rely on partners or friends for support, rather than their biological family members (for a good overview of these dynamics see Allen and Roberto 2016).

Senior living staff have a unique opportunity to integrate a resident's chosen family into the community, help the family of origin adjust to this new information, and form stronger relationships. In some cases, they may even need to protect LGBT people from members of their family of origin who may not have their best interests at heart.

FAMILIES OF CHOICE IN RESIDENTIAL COMMUNITIES

A vibrant residential community is not a monastery or a retreat—it's a social hub with visitors coming and going all day long. Many communities have family visiting events and encourage family members to be an active part of a resident's life. How can staff encourage both families of origin and families of choice to be an active part of the community, and how can these families help to enhance the quality of life for residents?

The first step is to make sure that when you mention family or welcoming families you do not inadvertently send the message that family means heterosexual or non-LGBT families only.

Terms like "family values" and anti-LGBT groups with names like Focus on the Family have created a negative association for many LGBT people, and if mention of family is accompanied by pictures of non-LGBT people, it may communicate that LGBT people are not present or welcome in the community.

One simple way to avoid this is to always include the phrase "all families welcome" on promotional materials or to be clear that activities are open to all by saying things like, "You can bring family members, significant others, friends, or other important people to your care planning meeting." Similar to our discussion of open-ended questions in Chapter 2, taking the extra time to expand on your definition of family can make it clear to LGBT people that they can bring anyone in their family of choice or support network. Another change is to use inclusive imagery. Photographs of LGBT families, groups of friends, and other groupings of people help send an inclusive message. If you are planning something like a family day, avoid images of heterosexual families and instead use neutral icons such as a picnic basket or an open doorway.

Once a person's family of choice has started to visit, it's important that staff treat them with the same respect and warmth that they would a person's biological or legal relations. The visitor may be introduced as a "friend," but that may be a euphemism, and even if it is not, no matter how the people define their relationship that visitor deserves the same level of courtesy as the most involved biological son or daughter.

If someone is being cared for by a large network of people—perhaps members of an LGBT center's friendly visitor program—staff may be interacting with many different people, which might be strange for staff who are more used to working with a handful of family members for each resident. Some staff may find it odd that ten different people from the LGBT community center visit each month, but in reality this is no different than volunteers from a church or a resident's social circle dropping by. This is where a resident's file can be a useful tool, as staff can record the names of frequent visitors as well as how they describe their relationship with the resident. By doing so, staff—especially across shift changes—can be aware of who is in the community and the best way to understand their relationships with the resident.

You can fully integrate a resident's partner, family of choice, and other support systems into a resident's life without that resident ever needing to come out to you as LGBT. If you think that a resident's visitor is their partner but they describe themselves as friends, make sure the resident knows that their friend or anyone else can be their power of attorney. Likewise, the nurses may know that the volunteer visitor is from an LGBT community group, but they can simply announce that "your visitor is here" and make them feel welcome, without forcing either person to disclose that they met at an LGBT center. As the residents and visitors become more comfortable they may decide to come out, but staff can achieve the goals of protecting the resident's wishes and supporting their caregivers without anybody feeling pressured to discuss being LGBT. As always, the key is to create a sense of safety, reflect back the language you are hearing, and let people move at their own pace.

BOX 7.2 CASE STUDY

How to integrate families of choice into long-term care networks

Objectives

- Identify the challenges of identifying an appropriate LGBT-friendly long-term care environment for individuals with dementia.
- Discuss useful strategies to successfully integrate families of choice into the care community.
- List opportunities for organizational change and business development related to LGBT-competent and sensitive care.

Introduction

Mark is a 66-year-old gay male, diagnosed five years ago with frontotemporal dementia (FTD). He has been in a loving and committed relationship with Steven for 35 years. They lived in a city high-rise condo until Mark became more symptomatic with increasingly impaired decision-making skills, impulsive behavior, need for assistance with showering and dressing, and frequent falls.

Relevant background and social history

Mark was forced to retire from teaching high-school English six years ago due to problems planning and organizing lectures and grades. Steven, age 57, works full time as a sociology professor at a local community college. They have a strong core circle of four supportive LGBT friends—their *family of choice*. The couple can no longer afford increasing out-of-pocket expenses for paid companion services. Mark and Steven have been estranged from their families of origin for the past 20 years. Mark enjoys theater, singing in choirs, and traveling.

The search for a long-term care environment was narrowed by the following criteria: memory care support, accepts Medicare/Medicaid, maximum 15 miles' distance from Steven's work. Two communities resulted; the hope for an LGBT-friendly environment would be a bonus. Only one of the two communities listed a non-discrimination policy regarding sexual orientation. Eighteen women and four men with middle to late stages of dementia resided within the selected memory care community.

Challenging issues related to LGBT identify and care

From admission through the first two months, there was a mix of subtle and blatant care concerns exposing the need for improvements in sensitivity, education, competency, staffing, and policy.

- Documents, consents, charting options were based upon heterosexual relationships.
- Brochures and marketing information with a majority of images with white heterosexual couples with grandchildren.
- Staff hesitant to engage or listen to concerns from Mark's core *family of choice*.
- Steven sensed the staff's discomfort when he held Mark's hand or kissed him goodbye in the community living room.
- Because of inconsistent staffing patterns and use of temporary agency personnel, some staff assumed that Mark had multiple partners when any *family of choice* members would visit.

After three months, Mark started to masturbate almost daily during afternoon activity sessions. Staff tried to deter him with loud and shaming requests to stop. This hypersexuality is a fairly common experience with individuals diagnosed with FTD. It is related to changes in regulating executive functioning impulse control. Unfortunately, the staff was not as well versed in the characteristics of FTD as expected and assumed this was an expression of his "homosexuality." Steven refused the memory care manager's request to use an antipsychotic medication to control the behavior.

Steps to address challenges and concerns

Requested a care plan meeting with the unit manager, Mark's care team, Steven, and *family of choice* to address

- Non-drug strategies to minimize hypersexuality.

  - Provided overview of FTD and its unique characteristics. Explained that hypersexuality is not connected to Mark's sexual orientation.
  - Identified potential triggers for Mark's hypersexual behavior: lack of engagement in meaningful activities, anxiety and boredom.
  - Instructed staff on how to distract with conversation and new activities in a respectful manner.
  - Coached activity manager to integrate person-centered programming related to Mark's enjoyment of singing and theatre.

- Integration of sensitive and competent LGBT care.

  - Discussed meaning and importance of *family of choice.*
  - Requested that names, contact info, and photos of members within Mark's *family of choice* be placed in the chart and care plan.
  - Met separately with executive director, health administrator, and director of nursing with suggested strategies to make the environment more LGBT-welcoming.

    - Revise intake, consents, and other forms to be LGBT-inclusive.
    - Include LGBT non-discrimination policies and recognizable logos on their website, entry ways.
    - Include photos of LGBT elders in their marketing materials.
    - Hire LGBT staff.
    - If agreed to by Mark's power of attorney, include members within the *family of choice* in care plan sessions.
    - Invite *family of choice* members to family council committees.
    - Require LGBT sensitivity training for all clinical, administrative, and non-clinical employees.
    - Incorporate Pride week information, history, and activities during June.
    - Add LGBT-focused questions to family and staff satisfaction surveys.
    - Add LGBT care competencies and criteria within job descriptions and performance reviews.
    - Provide references to LGBT websites for further assistance.

Progress thus far

- Mark's hypersexual behavior stopped entirely once music and singing were included routinely in scheduled activities. Staff learned to start asking Mark about his favorite Broadway shows if he showed signs of boredom or anxiety.
- Members with Mark's *family of choice* report being frequently referred to as his *"family"* and addressed with more friendly and genuine conversations by direct care staff.
- Facilitated a discussion and learning circle on LGBT sensitive language and care for residents with and without dementia with the goal of including this information in the educational required curriculum for all of their facilities.
- Steven is much more comfortable holding Mark's hand as they sit together in the living room or walk together throughout the household.
- Everything else is a work in progress.

Jeannine Forrest, Ph.D., R.N.
Dementia Educator and Care Consultant
Through the Forrest
www.throughtheforrest.com

CONFLICT WITHIN FAMILIES OF ORIGIN

Unfortunately, it may be the case that an older adult's family of origin is not at all involved but appears periodically, or re-enters the scene when the resident is nearing the end of life. Some family members may be seeking genuine reconciliation, others may be feeling guilt, or perhaps they want to be sure they get the family jewelry.

Whatever their motivations, this can lead to conflict, especially when members of the resident's family of origin do not accept their LGBT identity or do not respect the resident's family of choice. Here are some of the scenarios I have encountered over the years:

- The family of origin does not accept the same-sex partner and refuses to let them visit the resident.
- The family of origin does not accept their parent's gender identity and refuses to respect their name, pronouns, or gender expression.
- The family of origin moves the resident to a new community, often isolating the resident from chosen family and other supports.
- The family of origin refuses to let the resident's family of choice visit or participate in decision-making.

As I detail in Chapter 12, advanced directives are an important way to help a resident establish who can and cannot make decisions on their behalf, as well as protecting their partner or other chosen family in the event that the resident becomes incapacitated or dies. This is why the first conversations when a resident moves into your community are crucially important. If an LGBT resident has strained relations with their family of origin, questions like "Are you married?" or "Do you have kids?" may get a one- or two-word response, whereas a statement like "Tell me about yourself and your community" invites the resident to describe their family of choice. Likewise, conversations around surrogate decision-makers and a resident's preferences around their grooming and gender expression, as well as who they do and do not want to visit, are all important ways to give staff the information they need to advocate for the resident's interests.

If a resident is openly LGBT in your community but is not out to their family of origin, it is important to communicate with the resident to make sure that staff and other residents know how to behave when the family visits, what terms to use, how to interact with the resident, and in the case of transgender residents, which names and pronouns to use when the family is present. Ideally, all people involved would feel comfortable being open, but if a resident is not ready to have these conversations with their family, that is their choice. Similarly, if they do want to come out to family your staff can provide support, mediation, and resources and create a safe space for that resident to come to terms with coming out.

The primary concern is making sure the resident's wishes are being followed. This may upset the family, but explaining to them that it is your responsibility to advocate for the resident sets an important baseline expectation. If a biological family member is the legal decision-maker they may need help understanding how to do what is best for the resident, especially if it makes the family member uncomfortable. For example, they may not want their father to be romantic with another man, and staff can work with the family to help them see the positive impact the relationship has for their parent. If there continues to be conflict between the resident's wishes or behaviors and the family, consider bringing in your local ombudsman. Their job is to advocate for the resident's rights, and as an outside voice it may take some of the attention away from staff and allow them to continue focusing on the resident while also providing support to the family.

Family members may be experiencing guilt or surprise, and providing them with resources like support groups, meeting with a social worker, and connecting them to a local PFLAG chapter may ease their own feelings of confusion or discomfort. For more information on family reactions to resident sexual behavior see Chapter 8, and for information on protecting a resident's wishes when they have dementia or declining health see Chapter 12.

IT TAKES A VILLAGE

Family can mean many things, and each of us needs to feel situated within a network of trusted individuals in order to flourish. This chapter described what can be unique about an LGBT resident's family of choice, but it must be taken in tandem with the other chapters in this book if staff are going to have the skills they need to navigate the difficult and emotional questions that can be raised by both families of origin and chosen families.

SUGGESTIONS

- Ask open-ended questions to discover your resident's care network, paying special attention to people who are not biological or legal family, and asking appropriate follow-up questions.
- When things become heated remember that your first and primary responsibility is to advocate for the resident.
- Remember that family members may lash out due to stress or guilt. Try to determine if their complaint has roots that are deeper than the issue at hand, and offer suggestions for connecting with local support groups and resources.
- Utilize advanced directives and legal protections to ensure that your resident's wishes are followed and to protect their partner or chosen family members.

FURTHER READING AND VIEWING

Brennan-Ing, M. Seidel, L. Larson, B. & Karpiak, S. E. 2014. "Social Care Networks and LGBT Older Adults: Challenges for the Future." *Journal of Homosexuality* 61 (1): 21–52.
"Caregiving in the LGBT Community: A Guide to Engaging and Supporting LGBT Caregivers through Programming" (www.lgbtagingcenter.org).
Croghan, C.F. Moone, R.P., & Olson, A.M. 2014. "Family, Friends, Caregiving among Midlife and Older Lesbian, Gay, Bisexual, and Transgender Adults." *Journal of Homosexuality* 61 (1): 79–102.
"PFLAG—A Support Network for Parents and Friends of LGBT People." (www.pflag.org).
"Prepare to Care: A Planning Guide for Caregivers in the LGBT Community" (www.sageusa. org/).

REFERENCES

Allen, Katherine R., and Karen A. Roberto. 2016. "Family Relationships of Older LGBT Adults." In *Handbook of LGBT Elders*, edited by Debra A. Harley and Pamela B. Teaster, 43–64. Cham: Springer International Publishing. https://doi.org/10.1007/978-3-319-03623-6.

8

SEXUALITY AND SEXUAL HEALTH

SUMMARY

Sexual expression is a healthy part of the human experience and an important way to feel connected and affirmed, at any age. This chapter begins by explaining that discussing sexual orientation is not the same thing as discussing sexual activity. After making this distinction the chapter discusses how to support all people, including those engaging in same-sex or non-traditional sexual relationships, in their right to sexual expression while also respecting your staff's right to be free from mistreatment and sexual harassment.

OBJECTIVES

- Identify the importance of sexual expression for people of all ages and the unique barriers faced by those interested in same-sex sexual activity or engaging in relationships other than monogamous heterosexuality.
- Learn how to support residents who want to engage in consensual sexual activity.
- Discuss how to set clear boundaries and prevent inappropriate sexual behavior or sexual harassment.

AGING DOESN'T STOP DESIRE!

What do the words "sex symbol" bring to mind? For most of us, when we picture a sexy person we think of someone young, with a toned body and confident energy. Our society often pairs youth with sex, and one impact of ageism is that it de-sexualizes older people. Stereotypes of older adults can be negative or positive, with cranky old men and cat ladies on the one hand, and wise elder statesmen and sweet grandmothers on the other, but rarely are those stereotypes sexy. Yes, there are some terms, like "silver fox" or "cougar," that describe older people as sexy and sexually active, but a silver fox or cougar on television is probably in their mid-40s or early 50s, not their 70s, 80s, or 90s.

As a result, many staff never consider that residents have sexual desires or sex lives and may react poorly or with negative feelings, or be unsure how to react, when they see evidence of residents' sexual activity (Grigorovich and Kontos 2016). This unwillingness to discuss sexuality can create several negative outcomes. First, by not discussing sexuality and sexual expression older adults may not have access to information they need to have safer sex. Some older people may think, incorrectly, that because they cannot become pregnant there is no need to use condoms, dental dams, and other barriers. This lack of education has led to high rates of sexually transmitted infections in a variety of senior living environments. Data comparing 2015 to 2016 shows a 20 percent increase in sexually transmitted infections among older people (Lilleston n.d.). In addition, many providers have the misperception that older adults do not use illicit drugs, and drug use can increase the risk of transmitting sexually transmitted infections (Davis and Sokan 2016, 393–4).

Second, if we do not discuss sexuality and sexual expression, residents may not feel empowered to seek out and pursue sexual relationships. Closing off this aspect of the human experience can diminish their quality of life and lead to feelings of disconnectedness and isolation.

Third, without frank discussions about sexuality, staff may continue to confuse sexual orientation (who someone is attracted to) with sexual expression or activity, making it harder to discuss the unique needs of lesbian, gay, and bisexual older people.

For these reasons and more it is important to openly discuss sex and sexuality in our communities.

SEXUAL ORIENTATION IS DIFFERENT FROM SEXUAL ACTIVITY

It is important that residents can discuss both their sexual activity and their sexual orientation, but we must not confuse these two aspects of the human experience. When I train staff and suggest that they ask questions about a resident's sexual orientation or consider how a person's sexual orientation is a part of their history, I often see at least one person look confused and then a little agitated. After several minutes they will raise their hand and say something like, "I could never ask our residents what they do in bed!"

This sentiment reflects an understandable and common misconception that discussing a person's sexual orientation—who they are attracted to physically, emotionally, and intellectually—is the same thing as asking what they do in bed, which we call "sexual expression" or "sexual activity." If you think about it, we discuss our orientations all the time without disclosing anything about sexual expression. If I attend a wedding for a man and woman, that ceremony is in part an expression of their straight or perhaps bisexual identities, but it does not tell me anything about how they express or act on their sexual desires. Likewise, I can come out as a gay man without telling anyone anything about what I like to do in bed.

As noted previously, it is important that residents feel comfortable discussing sexual expression in an appropriate manner. They may need access to erotic materials, lubrication or toys, or preventative education and supplies and have concerns about their relationship or need to find a place to discuss the different meanings of sex and intimacy as they grow older.

On the other hand, knowing about a resident's sexual orientation can tell you a lot about their experience and personal history. As we have discussed in previous chapters, if a resident cannot disclose their sexual orientation they will be forced to hide aspects of their past, their relationships, or their current community.

These are two important but very different conversations—and it may be the case that a resident is comfortable talking about their sexual orientation but chooses to remain private about their sexual activity.

SEXUAL EXPRESSION IN RESIDENTIAL SETTINGS

Spend a minute in a resident's shoes. Ilana is a woman living in a community with very little privacy. Her meals and social activities are spent with the same people each day, and she often needs help with everyday tasks. Ilana and her neighbor Julia are attracted to each other, and she would like to spend some intimate time together, but she also knows that staff often enter rooms without knocking, and she is concerned about other residents gossiping or treating her badly because she is attracted to another woman.

This is a frustrating situation for these two women, and without support they might simply deny themselves the desire for intimacy and physical contact. Staff have a unique opportunity to help ensure that doesn't happen, that these two people are able to express their sexual desires.

Of course, it would be easiest to take a totally hands-off approach, saying, "Whatever these two women do is their own business!"—but in this situation a hands-off approach fails to meet the residents' needs. While it is important to give people privacy, the women may have to discuss their sexual desires with staff in order to arrange for the privacy and assistance they need to be intimate and safe, such as allowing them to lock the door, helping the women dress and undress, or helping them get into and out of the bed. If the doors in your community do not have locks, find other ways for staff and residents to ensure that residents can have time together without disturbance.

In this scenario, because the women are afraid of staff or other residents treating them poorly, it is also important that both women can talk to trusted staff about their same-sex attraction. Staff can help support the women in the ways described here and also by setting expectations in the community that their relationship will be respected, not ridiculed.

These two women may be sexually attracted to each other but not identify as lesbian or bisexual. They may be experiencing these attractions but not want to take on the identity or label. Talking about a person's identity is not always the same thing as discussing their behavior, and vice-versa. It is possible to talk about a resident identifying as lesbian, gay, or bisexual and not get into any discussion about sexual behavior, and it is possible to support a resident's sexual expression without making assumptions about how they identify.

CREATING A SEX POSITIVE ATMOSPHERE

The phrase "sex positive" may seem a little extreme or out of place in a senior living community, but what I mean by "sex positive" is creating an environment where people feel comfortable discussing sex and sexuality within appropriate boundaries.

Many times, when staff or administrators see sexual behavior they are primarily concerned with safety, how family members will react, or the fear of a lawsuit. While these can all be legitimate concerns, it is important to recognize that older adults have the right to express themselves sexually, and their behavior must be understood in the context of both their specific relationships and the wider community (Doll 2012; Grigorovich and Kontos 2016). It is beyond the scope of this book to address all of the ways to create a sex positive community, but consider some general recommendations:

- Ensure residents have the space, privacy, and help necessary to express their sexuality.
- Train staff to always knock when entering a closed room or home.
- Provide residents with access to erotic materials, preventative barriers including external and internal condoms, lubricants, and other sex aides.
- Establish a team of clinicians to monitor residents' ability to consent to sexual activity.
- Train staff on the signs of sexual assault or abuse.
- If you are medical staff taking a sexual history, include options beyond heterosexual sexual activity, and remember that sexual activity may not always align with sexual orientation or identity (for example, a man may have sex with other men but not identify as gay or bisexual).

Remember that stereotypes about race and religion also play into how we think about sex and sexuality. Erroneous beliefs that certain racial and ethnic groups are hypersexual while others are less sexual or submissive may influence how a particular resident's sexual behavior is assessed by staff. Each resident must be seen holistically, their sexual expression understood in the context of their identity, health, the relationship, and the wider community.

Finally, accepting and supporting sexuality between older adults does not mean creating a totally permissive, free-for-all atmosphere. Clear boundaries and expectations are an important part of a healthy culture, and residents and staff should always be protected from inappropriate touching, comments, or sexual harassment or assault. As discussed elsewhere throughout this book, members of the LGBT community, especially bisexual and transgender older adults, are disproportionately likely to be survivors of sexual assault. It is essential to train staff on how to identify, intervene, and report if they see signs of sexual assault or coercion. It is important that all people involved are able to affirmatively consent to sexual contact. If one or both residents have dementia a trained team of staff should constantly monitor their interactions. Consent and dementia is a complicated topic, but with proper staff involvement people living with dementia can continue to express themselves in an intimate setting. One good place to start is a white paper titled "Capacity for Sexual Consent in Dementia in Long-Term Care" from the Society for Post-Acute and Long-Term Care Medicine (available at https://paltc.org/), as well as some of the resources in Box 8.1.

BOX 8.1 ADDITIONAL RESOURCES TO SUPPORT SEXUAL EXPRESSION

The National Consumer Voice for Quality Long-Term Care has collected many resources on sexual expression and sexual abuse and assault. This page also includes the *Policies and Procedures Concerning Sexual Expression at The Hebrew Home at Riverdale*, which was one of the first and most influential policies adopted in the United States:
> http://ltcombudsman.org/issues/sexuality-and-intimacy-in-long-term-care-facilities:

The National Institute on Aging has collected a number of different resources on sexuality and dementia on their website, titled "Intimacy and Sexuality: Resources for Dementia Caregivers":
> www.nia.nih.gov/

The Alzheimer's Association also has fact sheets and supports on how Alzheimer's disease and other dementias can change sexuality and intimacy:
> www.alz.org

The impacts of aging, as well as chronic illness or pain, can change what it means to be sexually active. The ALS Society of Canada has produced a resource titled "Sexuality, Intimacy & Chronic Illness" that many residents may find helpful:
> www.als.ca/

Similarly, the American College of Rheumatology has resources on sexuality and arthritis:
> www.rheumatology.org/

Safer Sex for Seniors provides information and educational materials, including a humorous video introducing the topic of sexual expression between older adults:
> http://safersex4seniors.org

Age is Not a Condom is a prevention campaign specifically for older adults, and contains many LGBT-affirming images:
> http://ageisnotacondom.org/en/home/

Sex surrogacy is another way that individuals, pairs, or groups of people may express and enjoy their sexual desires. These therapists can use sexual expression to help individuals and couples have more satisfying and affirming sex lives and sexual expression, and can also help survivors of sexual assault and rape reconnect with sexual expression. Note: sexual surrogacy is not the same as sex work. For more information visit the International Professional Surrogates Association:
> www.surrogatetherapy.org

SPECIFIC CONCERNS FOR SAME-SEX SEXUAL CONTACT

There is a common belief or fear that long-term care staff will react more harshly or negatively to same-sex sexual contact than to heterosexual or different-sex interactions. One recent study found that many long-term care staff were supportive of older adults' sexuality and did not stigmatize same-sex sexual contact more than contact between different-sex couples (Ahrendt et al. 2017). However, the study surveyed a relatively small number of participants, was based on staff members' perceptions of their own reactions to a vignette, and transgender people were not included in the vignettes. Much more research is needed to determine if we are seeing a change in attitudes toward same-sex sexual contact in long-term care communities. A recent survey commissioned by GLAAD found that for the first time in years there has been a decrease in Americans' comfort with and acceptance of LGBT people generally (GLAAD 2018), so we all need to be aware that staff and residents may react to same-sex sexual relationships differently than they would different-sex couplings.

Whether or not LGBT people feel comfortable expressing their sexuality depends in large part on staff. Staff will always have feelings, opinions, and reactions to residents' sexual expression, which is fine. It is human nature to have opinions, and sexuality may be an uncomfortable topic. One's thoughts and feelings are not the problem; rather, the problem is unfair or negative actions, such as keeping same-sex couples apart or outing them without permission to their families or other residents.

Apart from gay and lesbian people, bisexual people face a number of unique stereotypes. The first is that bisexual people are more sexually active than other people. Some bisexual people may be very sexually active and others not at all, as is also the case with monosexual people (those only attracted to one gender). Second, some people assume that bisexuality is a phase, when in fact it is an identity and a genuine expression of a person's sexual orientation and desires. Finally, it is easy to erase bisexual identities by assuming that a person's current partner reflects the entirety of their sexual orientation. For example, two different-sex people in a couple are assumed to be straight, and the members of a same-sex couple are assumed to be gay or lesbian, when in both couples one or both partners may identify as bisexual. These stereotypes may influence how staff and other residents react to bisexual people in the community. For more information about bisexuality see Chapter 9.

Know that residents may start to explore new desires as they settle in to your community. For example, a man who has only ever had female partners might develop a romantic relationship with another male resident. This can be challenging if these behaviors are surprising or difficult for family members to understand. Chapter 7 explored navigating family reactions and emotions, and Chapter 12 discusses what happens when these changes are accompanied by dementia. The important thing to remember here is that as long as both residents consent to the sexual contact they should be allowed and empowered to pursue it, and the family does not need to be told unless there is a safety concern or legal reason to discuss their relationship.

BOX 8.2   INTERSECTION BETWEEN LGBT, MINORITY GROUPS, AND SEXUAL EXPRESSION: AN AUSTRALIAN PERSPECTIVE

Internationally, LGBT aging issues in developed countries have received growing attention with an increasing number of initiatives being introduced in the aging sectors to support older LGBT individuals. For example, in Australia, the Rainbow Tick Accreditation Program has been introduced to recognize organizations focused on providing LGBT-inclusive care and support in a safe and quality-focused environment (Quality Innovation Performance 2018). Australian academics together with LGBT advocates have called for an intersectional approach to recognize the diversity of social identities and lived experience and needs of older LGBT individuals. Specifically, the adoption of an intersectional lens to address the impact of multiple forms of discrimination on the health and wellbeing of older LGBT individuals who identify with other minority groups (e.g. Aboriginal) (Leonard and Mann 2018).

In recent times, research has begun to examine the interaction between (a) heterosexism and race and (b) ethnocentrism and ageism, as well as how it impacts on the health and wellbeing of vulnerable subpopulations within the LGBT communities (i.e. older age, minority and diverse cultural groups) (Leonard and Mann 2018). For instance, LGBT people of color reported higher incidences of receiving biased and inferior care than others (Lambda Legal 2010). However, there remains to be limited work on how multiple forms of discrimination affect the health and wellbeing of LGBT people within this growing body of work on "minorities within a minority" (Martino 2017; Leonard and Mann 2018).

One such area is sexual expression. Greater restrictions are placed on older LGBT people with intellectual and cognitive disabilities (e.g. dementia) where they are often regarded as either asexual or hypersexual, and if viewed as sexual, they are commonly considered heterosexual (Noonan and Gomez 2011; Wilson et al. 2016). There is also a dearth of available policies or programs that support older LGBT people's identities or promote their open and free sexual expression in an aged care environment (Leonard and Mann 2018). While it is encouraging to note the emergence of an intersectional lens in the development of policies and programs in Australia to assist older LGBT people with disabilities, and in some cases, those who identify with one or more other minority populations, gaps still exist, particularly when it comes to sexual expression in aged care. More research is needed to gain an understanding on how disparities in health outcomes among older LGBT people with disabilities and differences in sexual- and gender-diverse identity and expression are shaped and influenced by other categories of social inequality, such as race.

Given the precipitous change in demographics of Australia's older population, and even worldwide, it is timely to ruminate on and adopt an intersectional approach that takes into full consideration the differing social identities and life experiences and needs of older LGBT individuals. This is a helpful approach for care providers who are committed to tackling the sexual expression needs of older LGBT individuals with or without disability. Furthermore, besides leveraging the strengths and resiliencies of older LGBT individuals, this approach will stimulate social and policy progress by forming collaborative agendas and actions founded on the intersecting sexual expression needs and interests of older LGBT individuals.

Cindy Jones
Associate Professor of Behavioural Sciences
Faculty of Health Sciences & Medicine
Bond University, Queensland Australia

References

Lambda Legal. (2010). "When Health Care Isn't Caring: Lambda Legal's Survey of Discrimination against LGBT People and People Living with HIV." *Lambda Legal*. www.lambdalegal.org/publications/when-health-care-isnt-caring.

Leonard, W. and R. Mann. (2018) *The Everyday Experience of Lesbian, Gay, Bisexual, Transgender and Intersex (LGBTI) People Living with Disability*, No. 111 GLHV@ARCSHS, Melbourne: La Trobe University.

Martino, A.S. (2017). "Cripping Sexualities: An Analytic Review of Theoretical and Empirical Writing on the Intersection of Disabilities and Sexualities." *Sociology Compass* 11: e12471. https://doi.org/10.1111/soc4.12471.

Noonan, A., and M. Gomez. (2011). "Who's Missing? Awareness of Lesbian, Gay, Bisexual and Transgender People with Intellectual Disability." *Sexuality and Disability* 29 (2): 175–180.

Quality Innovation Performance. (2018). "Rainbow Tick Standards." *QIP*. www.qip.com.au/standards/rainbow-tick-standards/.

Wilson, N.J., A.M. Bright, J. Macdonald, P. Frawley, B. Hayman, and G. Gallego. (2016). "Narrative Review of the Literature about People with Intellectual Disability who Identity as Lesbian, Gay, Bisexual, Transgender, Intersex or Questioning." *Journal of Intellectual Disabilities*: 1–26. https://doi.org/10.1177/1744629516682681.

OTHER WAYS TO HAVE RELATIONSHIPS

Many older adults hold the traditional view that monogamous relationships are best, or that sexual activity should only take place between married people. That said, just as what it means to have sex and be intimate can change with age, so too can the kinds of relationships people desire. A person may be non-monogamous or in an open relationship where all people involved understand they are not exclusive, or two people may be monogamous but not be married, not live together, and maintain very independent lives.

Intimacy does not always involve sexual expression. Two people can be in a committed relationship without engaging in sexual activity. For example, two women may live together, share a deep commitment to one another's lives, and perhaps be physically affectionate but not identify as lesbian or bisexual and not have a sexual relationship. This could be confusing for staff, who may assume that the women are hiding the nature of their relationship by saying they are friends or roommates. This further emphasizes the importance of not making assumptions about how people define their relationships, but rather creating the environment and culture where their relationships can be affirmed and protected in whatever way the residents desire.

Each relationship is as unique as the people in it and may not fit within the expectations of staff or other residents. The most important thing to do is make sure people are safe, empowered, and given the privacy they need to seek out whatever types of relationships they desire.

SUGGESTIONS

■ Recognize that all residents have the right to consensual sexual contact and that if someone engages in same-sex sexual contact they are not necessarily confused or being taken advantage of, but in fact may be expressing a new or previously hidden desire.
■ Understand that sex means different things to different people and changes as we age.
■ Remember that discussion of a person's LGBT identity is about their history, culture, and relationships and is different than discussing sexual behavior.
■ Draw clear professional boundaries to protect staff from unwanted sexual advances.

FURTHER READING AND VIEWING

Ageing and Sexualities: Interdisciplinary Perspectives, edited by Elizabeth Peel and Rosie Harding.
Beauty Before Age: Growing Older in Gay Culture (film).
"Intimacy and Sexuality: Resources for Dementia Caregivers" (www.nia.nih.gov/).
"Safer Sex for Seniors" (http://safersex4seniors.org).
Sexuality and Long-Term Care: Understanding and Supporting the Needs of Older Adults by Gay Appel Doll.

REFERENCES

Ahrendt, Andrew, Eric Sprankle, Alex Kuka, and Keagan McPherson. 2017. "Staff Member Reactions to Same-Gender, Resident-to-Resident Sexual Behavior Within Long-Term Care Facilities." *Journal of Homosexuality* 64 (11): 1502–18. https://doi.org/10.1080/00918369.2016.1247533.

Davis, Tracy, and Amanda Sokan. 2016. "Healthcare, Sexual Practices, and Cultural Competence with LGBT Elders." In *Handbook of LGBT Elders*, edited by Debra A. Harley and Pamela B. Teaster, 391–415. Cham: Springer International Publishing. https://doi.org/10.1007/978-3-319-03623-6.

Doll, Gayle Appel. 2012. *Sexuality & Long-Term Care: Understanding and Supporting the Needs of Older Adults*. Baltimore, MD: Health Professions Press.

GLAAD. 2018. "Accelerating Acceptance 2018: A Survey of American Acceptance and Attitudes Toward LGBTQ Americans, Executive Summary." *GLAAD*. www.glaad.org/files/aa/Accelerating%20Acceptance%202018.pdf.

Grigorovich, Alisa, and Pia Kontos. 2016. "Advancing an Ethic of Embodied Relational Sexuality to Guide Decision-Making in Dementia Care." *The Gerontologist* 58 (2): 219–25. https://doi.org/10.1093/geront/gnw137.

Lilleston, Randy. n.d. "STD Rates Continue to Rise for Older Adults." *AARP*. Accessed September 9, 2018. www.aarp.org/health/conditions-treatments/info-2017/std-exposure-rises-older-adults-fd.html.

9

BISEXUALITY AND AGING

SUMMARY

Some estimates indicate that there are twice as many bisexual people as there are gay and lesbian people. This may be surprising because bisexual people are often an invisible part of both the LGBT and non-LGBT communities. This chapter explores what you and your team can do to create environments where bisexual people are affirmed, help spot and prevent bias against bisexual people, and consider what is unique about aging as a bisexual person.

OBJECTIVES

- Dispel common myths about bisexual people.
- Learn how our assumptions may make bisexual older adults invisible and delegitimize their identities.
- Consider the differences between the life experiences of a gay or lesbian person and a bisexual person, including the impact of being bisexual on family structure and relationships.

BISEXUALITY DEFINED

There are a number of ways to define bisexuality, with the most common definition being that a bisexual is someone who is attracted to both men and women. Not everyone is comfortable with this definition because it may imply that bisexual people are equally attracted to men and women, or that there are only two genders. Bisexual activist and educator Robyn Ochs says this about her bisexuality:

> I call myself bisexual because I acknowledge in myself the potential to be attracted—romantically and/or sexually—to people of more than one sex and/or gender, not necessarily at the same time, in the same way, or to the same degree.
>
> (Ochs n.d.)

This definition is expansive and captures a broader range of bisexual experiences, and it also recognizes that the kind or degree of attraction someone feels may change over a lifetime.

Some people do not use the term "bisexual" because the prefix "bi-" implies that there are only two genders. This can carry a negative association for people whose gender identity is fluid, different from either male or female, for some transgender, intersex, gender nonconforming or genderqueer individuals, or for someone who is attracted to people with those gender identities. The term "pansexual" (the prefix "pan-" means "all" or "everything") describes attraction to people of multiple genders. Some bisexual people may experience attraction to people who identify as non-binary or transgender, but continue to use the term "bisexual" because it is a term they feel comfortable with and are accustomed to using. Many people also use the word "queer" to describe their sexual orientation, which can be a more expansive way to describe a sexual orientation other than heterosexual.

As always, the most important things are to remember and reflect whatever word a person prefers to use to describe their identity and not to make assumptions based on their current or past relationships.

THE INVISIBLE MAJORITY

Many people are surprised to learn that bisexual people make up more than half of the adult LGB population, that people of color are more likely to identify as bisexual than white people, and that while older adults are somewhat less likely to identify as bisexual they are still a large part of the LGB community (MAP 2016). When compared to lesbian and gay people, bisexual people are less likely to be out to the important people in their lives, and bisexual people over 45 are less likely to be out to those important people than bisexual people under 45 years of age (Parker 2013). There are many reasons why, despite being such a large part of the LGBT community, bisexual people are often invisible.

First, people often make assumptions about a person's sexual orientation based on their current relationship. Two men together are assumed to be gay, two women are assumed to be lesbians, and a man and women are seen as heterosexual. Many people do not stop to consider that one or both of the people in a couple may be bisexual, pansexual, or queer. If a woman is married to a man and after her divorce starts dating a woman, it is easy to assume they divorced because she was closeted and is now an out lesbian. However, if the woman has always identified as bisexual that narrative would be incorrect, and treating her with respect requires not jumping to any conclusions about how she identifies.

There are generational differences, as well. "Queer" is becoming a more common word to describe people with multiple attractions or indicate a sexual orientation other that heterosexual, and older bisexual folks may or may not find that word affirming. Some older adults may have spent years identifying as gay or lesbian and may now be feeling attractions to people of a different gender and struggle with how to understand and communicate that desire. We tend to think of coming out as a change from identifying as straight to identifying as lesbian, gay, or bisexual—but I've known people who identified as gay or lesbian for decades and are now coming out as bisexual, and may be struggling to have that identify affirmed by their gay and lesbian communities.

Another reason bisexual people are invisible is that there are negative stereotypes about bisexual people both within and outside of the LGBT community. These include the incorrect belief that bisexual people are more sexually active than monosexual people (those only attracted to one gender, such as heterosexual, gay, or lesbian people), are less faithful or trustworthy, or are just "going through a phase." During the HIV/AIDS crisis, many bisexual men were blamed for transmitting HIV and other sexually transmitted infections from gay communities into the heterosexual population (Eliason 2000). Many people incorrectly think that bisexual people are equally attracted to both genders and that those who may have more attractions for a certain gender identity, or who are monogamous, are not really bisexual. These negative stereotypes all share the same core belief that bisexual people are not trustworthy or faithful, or that they just need to make up their minds.

Bisexual people face these stereotypes not only in the broader culture, but also inside the LGBT community. I have heard many gay and lesbian people accuse bisexual people of "wanting it both ways" or implying that they are not brave enough to fully come out. Bisexual people are also seen as benefitting from heterosexual privilege or passing as straight when it is convenient. The fact is, being openly bisexual is quite difficult, especially when faced with hostility within the LGBT community, which is why many people stay closeted about their bisexuality.

Finally, bisexual people are underrepresented in the media and politics, including in how we tell the story of the LGBT movement and the history of bisexual activism. Thankfully this is changing, and there are a growing number of notable public figures who are open about their bisexuality or queer orientation, or having partners of multiple genders, such as Alicia Garza, one of the founders of #BlackLivesMatter, who identifies as queer; Kate Brown, the governor of Oregon; David Bowie; and Lady Gaga, to name a few. That said, there are very few examples of out bisexual older adults in public life or in the media, and many characters who do display attractions to multiple genders may be portrayed as fluid or experimenting, and they do not explicitly identify as bisexual. For an overview and elaboration of these topics, specifically as it relates to bisexual older adults, see Scherrer 2017.

IMPACTS OF BIPHOBIA ACROSS THE LIFESPAN

Bi-invisibility and biphobia, both from those within and outside of the LGBT community, have real impacts on the health and wellbeing of bisexual older adults. One study found that 46.7 percent and 48.2 percent of bisexual older men and women respectively live at or below 200 percent of the federal poverty line (Emlet 2016). Bisexual older people with the same education level as their gay and lesbian peers make less money than gay and lesbian people and heterosexuals. Bisexual older people have worse physical and mental health than their gay, lesbian, and heterosexual peers (Fredriksen-Goldsen et al. 2016), and a recent study of bisexual people over 50 found that over an 18-year period they were less likely to report a positive change in life satisfaction than lesbian, gay, and heterosexual counterparts (Wardecker et al. 2018). Much of the research about bisexuality does not report specifically on bisexual people of color, who remain more marginalized and less visible within the category of bisexuality (Ghabrial and Ross 2018).

These disparities mean that bisexual seniors may have fewer financial resources, be experiencing health problems at a higher rate than other older adults, and have faced significant discrimination and bias. Gender stereotypes also play into how people interact with bisexual people. Women are often seen as being more sexually fluid than men, and bisexual women may have a history of being fetishized or sexualized while bisexual men feel pressure to conform to masculine stereotypes that often do not allow for expressing same-sex sexual desire.

Lest I focus too much on the negative, as we have noted in other discussions of disparities, it is important to know the burdens faced by bisexual older adults, but we can also focus on their resiliency. The experiences of bisexual people can teach us a lot about being perceived as both heterosexual and as members of the LGBT community, and doing the work of becoming more sensitive to bisexual cultural competency is an opportunity to question our monosexist assumptions about ourselves and others.

AVOIDING ASSUMPTIONS AND AFFIRMING BISEXUALITY

Many bisexual people are monogamous and in long-term relationships. So when you meet a different-sex or same-sex couple it is important to remember that one or more people in that couple might identify as bisexual.

Many gay and lesbian seniors were married to different-sex partners and came out later in life. This is a common experience, but it is somewhat different for a bisexual person. As I noted previously, the typical narrative is that a person is in a heterosexual marriage and then comes out to live their authentic life. This narrative of hidden authenticity may not apply to a bisexual person who has always been open about their bisexuality with their monogamous partner, and in such cases wrongly implies that one relationship is more authentic than the other. It can also be the case that a resident has had sexual relationships with people of different genders at some point in their life, but never identified as a bisexual.

There is emerging evidence that at least among younger generations bisexual people are more likely than gay and lesbian people to have children or be parents. A report from the Williams Institute found that 59 percent of bisexual women and 32 percent of bisexual men had children, compared to 31 percent of lesbians and 16 percent of gay men, and nearly two thirds of LGB people who are parents are bisexual (Goldberg, Gartrell, and Gates 2014). This means that your bisexual residents are more likely to be navigating dynamics that include children, and if they have historically been in different-sex relationships their children may not know about their bisexuality or same-sex attractions. We often assume that people with children are heterosexual and/or cisgender, so it is important that staff are aware of the fact that many LGBT people, and especially bisexual people, are also parents. Chapter 7 gives an overview of how to navigate some of these family dynamics, and Chapter 12 provides advice for supporting residents with dementia who may be expressing desires that surprise their family members.

Another simple change you can make to increase bi-visibility is to watch out for moments when language erases bisexual people—for example, saying "gay" as an umbrella term instead of "LGBT," or saying "gay marriage" rather than "same-sex marriage." The first erases the visibility of bisexual and transgender people (as well as women who prefer the term "lesbian"), and the second implies that all people in same-sex marriages identify as gay or lesbian. These may sound like small things, but they can have an impact, especially when repeated over time. I see this happen during LGBT cultural competency trainings as well, so when selecting a training program be sure to review it and make sure that the content and facilitator can both speak to the perspectives of the bisexual community. For some common misconceptions and suggestions for addressing them during cultural competency trainings see Johnston 2016.

Remember that when you create LGBT-affirming programming, bisexual residents may not feel particularly welcome in LGBT spaces, and may perceive the spaces and programming as primarily geared toward gay and lesbian people. Consider explicitly celebrating Bisexual Awareness Month in March or Celebrate Bisexuality Day on September 23rd, and use bisexual-affirming imagery such as the bisexual pride flag (which is pink and blue with a horizontal purple stripe in the middle). When you are planning general LGBT Pride or history activities, be sure to include bisexual voices, topics, histories, and representation. If you hear anyone, even other LGBT residents, saying things that are disrespectful to bisexual people you can use it as an opportunity to educate them about the realities of bisexual peoples' lives and the importance of supporting bi-visibility.

As is the case with many of the terms and concepts in this book, what it means to be bisexual is in part a personal matter, and each person has their own understanding of what the term means to them. At the end of the day the most important thing is to treat each resident according to a person-centered approach and let them tell you about their life and identity.

BOX 9.1   A VIGNETTE: MURIEL

Muriel is 78. When she was a girl she had a series of intense 'crushes' on older girls but she met her husband-to-be when she was 18 and quickly fell in love with him. They got married and had three children. When Muriel was in her early-30s, her husband divorced her.

When she was in her late-30s Muriel joined a women's consciousness-raising group. In the group she came across the idea of lesbianism, which she had never heard discussed before and she met a woman, Pat, who already identified as a lesbian. Muriel was strongly attracted to her and before long they had started a relationship. After Muriel's children had left home, they lived together for several years, and became a familiar couple on the local lesbian scene. Pat developed breast cancer and, after many difficult months, she died. Muriel got a lot of support from her circle of lesbian friends and from a local voluntary organisation which supported lesbians and gay men who had been bereaved.

Some months later, to her astonishment, she fell in love with a man, Colin. Her friends were very disapproving of her new relationship and gradually cut contact with her. The new relationship flourished, although Muriel recognised that she was still attracted to women too and missed her old circle of friends, especially as she was still grieving for Pat. She didn't feel able to keep using the bereavement service because she no longer seemed to count as a lesbian.

In the mid 1980s, Muriel came across the idea of 'bisexuality' and started calling herself bisexual. After some years, the relationship with Colin ended amicably and Muriel met another woman, Joan, and went back to thinking of herself as lesbian because that was Joan's identity and she expected this to be the final relationship of her life.

Last year Joan died and Muriel experienced some major health problems. She started receiving home care. She gets on well with one of her regular carers who asked her about the photos she had up around the house of her former partners. Muriel answers honestly but is horrified to discover later that her carer has spread malicious gossip among her colleagues about her past, saying that Muriel had been sexually predatory and promiscuous.

Reprinted with permission from Jones, Rebecca L. 2016. "Sexual Identity Labels and Their Implications in Later Life: The Case of Bisexuality." In *Ageing and Sexualities: Interdisciplinary Perspectives*, edited by Elizabeth Peel and Rosie Harding. Abingdon: Routledge.

Imagine that Muriel is moving into your community, and that this conversation with her carers took place with your staff.

Discussion questions

What barriers might Muriel face when trying to access support groups?
If you heard staff spreading rumors like this, how would you respond?

SUGGESTIONS

■ Do not assume that a person's partner reflects the entirety of their sexual orientation. Let people tell you how they describe their relationships, rather than labeling the relationships yourself.

■ Avoid using the word "gay" as a stand-in for "LGBT" or "same-sex." For example, saying "gay marriage" instead of "same-sex marriage" erases bisexual people who are in same-sex marriages.

■ Ensure that LGBT training content and sessions discuss bisexuality and the perspectives of bisexual older people.

■ Be intentional about celebrating bisexual history and the contributions of bisexual people to LGBT history.

FURTHER READING AND VIEWING

Anything that Moves Magazine (http://atm.silmemar.org).
Bi: Notes for a Bisexual Revolution by Shiri Eisner.
"BiNet USA" (www.binetusa.org).
"Bisexual Invisibility: Impacts and Recommendations" by the San Francisco Human Rights Commission LGBT Advisory Committee Bisexual Resource Center (www.biresource.org).

Getting Bi: Voices of Bisexuals Around the World by Robyn Ochs and Sarah Rowley.

No Longer Invisi(BI)le: 10 Bisexual Women of Color to Celebrate (www.qwoc.org/2013/03/
no-longer-invisibile-10-bisexual-women-of-color-to-celebrate-qwoctalk/).

REFERENCES

Eliason, Mickey. 2000. "Bi-Negativity: The Stigma Facing Bisexual Men." *Journal of Bisexuality* 1 (2–3): 137–54. https://doi.org/10.1300/J159v01n02_05.

Emlet, Charles A. 2016. "Social, Economic, and Health Disparities Among LGBT Older Adults." *Generations (San Francisco, Calif.)* 40 (2): 16–22.

Fredriksen-Goldsen, Karen I., Chengshi Shiu, Amanda E.B. Bryan, Jayn Goldsen, and Hyun-Jun Kim. 2016. "Health Equity and Aging of Bisexual Older Adults: Pathways of Risk and Resilience." *The Journals of Gerontology Series B: Psychological Sciences and Social Sciences*, 72 (3): 468–78. https://doi.org/10.1093/geronb/gbw120.

Ghabrial, Monica A., and Lori E. Ross. 2018. "Representation and Erasure of Bisexual People of Color: A Content Analysis of Quantitative Bisexual Mental Health Research." *Psychology of Sexual Orientation and Gender Diversity* 5 (2): 132–42. https://doi.org/10.1037/sgd0000286.

Goldberg, Abbie E., Nanette K. Gartrell, and Gary Gates. 2014. "Research Report on LGB-Parent Families." *The Williams Institute: UCLA School of Law.* http://williamsinstitute.law.ucla.edu/wp-content/uploads/lgb-parent-families-july-2014.pdf.

Johnston, Tim R. 2016. "Bisexual Aging and Cultural Competency Training: Responses to Five Common Misconceptions." *Journal of Bisexuality* 16 (1): 99–111. https://doi.org/10.1080/15299716.2015.1046629.

Jones, Rebecca L. 2016. "Sexual Identity Labels and Their Implications in Later Life: The Case of Bisexuality." In *Ageing and Sexualities: Interdisciplinary Perspectives*, edited by Elizabeth Peel and Rosie Harding, 99–100. Abingdon: Routledge.

MAP. 2016. "Invisible Majority: The Disparities Facing Bisexual People and How to Remedy Them." *The Movement Advancement Project (MAP).* www.lgbtmap.org/file/invisible-majority.pdf.

Ochs, Robyn. n.d. "Biography." *RobynOchs.com.* Accessed April 27, 2019. https://robynochs.com/biography/.

Parker, Kim. 2013. "Chapter 3: The Coming Out Experience. A Survey of LGBT Americans." *Pew Research Center.* www.pewsocialtrends.org/2013/06/13/chapter-3-the-coming-out-experience/.

Scherrer, Kristin S. 2017. "Stigma and Special Issues for Bisexual Older Adults." *Annual Review of Gerontology and Geriatrics* 37 (1): 43–57. https://doi.org/10.1891/0198-8794.37.43.

Wardecker, Britney M., Jes L. Matsick, Jennifer E. Graham-Engeland, and David M. Almeida. 2018. "Life Satisfaction Across Adulthood in Bisexual Men and Women: Findings from the Midlife in the United States (MIDUS) Study." *Archives of Sexual Behavior* (March). https://doi.org/10.1007/s10508-018-1151-5.

10

GENDER IDENTITY AND EXPRESSION

SUMMARY

We all express our genders through our bodies, mannerisms, voices, personal grooming, clothing, names, and the pronouns we use every day. Gender expression changes over the course of our lives, and an important part of living with dignity is feeling in control of how people perceive us. This chapter focuses on gender identity and expression in a senior living setting, in particular what staff can do to ensure that transgender, intersex, and gender nonconforming older adults can openly express their gender identities.

OBJECTIVES

- Appreciate that we all express our genders every day and transgender and gender nonconforming older adults face unique barriers to having their identities and gender expression respected and validated.
- Learn how to ask for a person's name and pronouns, and how to apologize if you accidently use the incorrect name or pronouns.
- Examine your policies around bathrooms, roommates, and other sex-segregated spaces to ensure they are safer for transgender residents.
- Discuss ways to advocate for transgender older adults, including at the spa, salon, barber, or with other residents.

GENDER IDENTITY AND GENDER EXPRESSION

Have you ever had the experience of answering the telephone and the caller using the wrong pronoun or gendered term, such as "sir" or "ma'am"? Have you approached somebody from behind and called "Excuse me, sir!" to get their attention and been embarrassed when the person turns and corrects you? These common experiences are usually embarrassing, and they demonstrate how easily and routinely we make assumptions about other people's gender identities. We might not notice how often we make these assumptions until we make a mistake or are corrected.

Gender identity is the gender a person identifies with or their deeply felt sense of being female, male, a combination of both, neither, or some other gender. Gender identity is something personal and internal, and it is different from gender expression. Gender expression is how we all communicate our gender identity through things like clothing, personal grooming, tone and pitch of voice, vocabulary, mannerisms, pronouns, and interests or hobbies.

The term "transgender" is an umbrella term that describes the experience of people whose gender identity does not match the sex they were assigned at birth. When each child is born they are assigned a sex, usually based on their genitals. If a baby has a vagina they are typically assigned female, and if a baby has a penis they are assigned male. I like the phrase "sex assigned a birth," rather than biological sex, because it helps us remember that none of us can choose the sex we are assigned; it is a decision made for us.

The prefix "trans-" means "to cross over," so "transgender" can be understood to mean someone whose identity is not on the same side as the sex they were assigned at birth or is not congruent with their sex assigned at birth. The term "transgender woman" or "trans woman" describes someone assigned male at birth but who identifies as a woman. "Transgender man" or "trans man" describes a person who was assigned female at birth but identifies as a man. In casual conversation many people shorten the word "transgender" to "trans" and will say "trans man" or "trans woman."

For other people, the sex that they were assigned at birth does match up or is congruent with their gender identity. One word that can describe people like that is "cisgender." The prefix "cis-" means "on the same side as," so if someone was assigned the sex male at birth, there is an "M" on his birth certificate, and he identifies as a man, he may identify as cisgender because his sex assigned at birth and gender identity match.

Another term you may hear is "transsexual." "Transsexual" is a term that some people use to describe a person who has had gender-affirming medical procedures, such as hormone therapy or gender affirmation surgery. Generally speaking, "transsexual" is used in a way similar to "transgender," but it is a term that to some is older or outdated and not as expansive as the term "transgender." "Transsexual" was also a term used more frequently in the past, so working with older people you may encounter folks who are more familiar with that term than "transgender.'

"Transgender" and "transition" or "transitioning" (which I discuss later on) are both respectful terms that staff can feel comfortable using. One important note is that "transgender" is an adjective, not a noun, so always say, "He/she/they are transgender" or, "They are a transgender man/woman/person." Never say just "a transgender" or "transgenders" because to many that is disrespectful or dehumanizing.

GENDERQUEER, GENDER NONCONFORMING, GENDER NON-BINARY, AND INTERSEX

The term "transgender" can imply that there are only two genders and that transgender people want to move from one gender into the other. However, for many this view is too simplistic, and terms like "genderqueer," "gender nonconforming," or "gender non-binary" seek to expand past the binary idea of gender (the idea that everyone is either a man or a woman). People who identify as genderqueer may not identify as masculine or feminine, may understand their gender to be fluid, or may not feel that they have a strong gender identification. People who say they are gender nonconforming identify in a way that does not match up with our social expectations of masculine and feminine people. Gender non-binary people identify outside of or across the gender binary. These are only three of the many other terms that can describe a person's gender—as always, the most important thing is to use whatever term a resident feels affirms their identity. Because these terms often have a very individual and personal meaning, if you hear a resident use one of these terms, you may ask, "Can you tell me more about what that term means to you?"

"Intersex" is an umbrella term for people born with genitals and other bodily characteristics that do not fit typical societal definitions or expectations of male or female bodies. Many different medical conditions can cause ambiguous genitalia. Some estimates put the number of intersex people at around 1 out of every 1500 to 2000 births (Accord Alliance n.d.), with other studies putting the number at 2 percent of live births (Blackless et al. 2000) on the high end and 0.018 percent on the low end (Sax 2002). Some prefer to avoid the term "intersex" and instead refer to these various medical conditions as Disorders of Sexual Development, or DSDs (which is a term that applies to the conditions, not to the people). Some intersex people later identify as transgender, others as intersex, and others as male or female or other gender identities. Many intersex people have been subjected to procedures called "genital normalization surgery" to make their genitals look like what society deems typical, often making it difficult to have children or experience sexual pleasure later in life. These surgeries were often performed when the person was an infant, and their diagnosis and the surgery was kept a secret. While these standards of treatment are changing, many intersex people have experienced trauma at the hands of doctors and other medical professionals and may be very distrusting of providers and avoid seeking medical care.

For the remainder of this chapter I am going to use the word "transgender" as an umbrella term to include people who experience some kind of difference between the sex they were assigned at birth and their gender identity, but it is important to always remember to accept and affirm whatever term a person uses to describe themselves and their gender.

LIVING AS A TRANSGENDER OLDER ADULT

Transgender people, especially transgender older adults and people of color, face higher rates of discrimination and marginalization than other members of the LGBT community. For example, a survey of LGBT older adults found that transgender respondents reported significantly higher rates of victimization (such as police misconduct or verbal or physical violence) when compared to lesbian, gay, or bisexual older adults (Fredriksen-Goldsen et al. 2011). Some surveys are beginning to suggest that transgender older adults face high rates of sexual assault and elder abuse (Cook-Daniels and munson 2010). For a comprehensive view of the experiences of transgender people (of all ages, including older respondents) see Grant et al. 2011 and James et al. 2016.

Many transgender older adults come out later in life, often after retiring, their children moving out of the house, divorce, or the death of a spouse. When a person comes out as transgender, it is important to note that their family and community also go through a kind of transition and will need time and support to understand and then honor the transgender person's identity. As I discuss in the following section, transitioning is never a single event, but a process that involves both the transgender person and the people around them.

TRANSITIONING

In the broadest sense, transitioning is when a person brings their gender identity more in line with their body, their gender expression, and how people see them in the world. There are several different ways in which a person may transition, including socially, medically, and legally. Many of the people I train are unsure of how to discuss a person's transition, and it is important to know that the terms "transition" and "transitioning" are considered respectful and appropriate terms and should be used instead of other euphemisms like "process," "the change," "sex change," or "when so-and-so became a man/woman," which implies that they were not a man or woman to begin with, which is not accurate.

Social transition

The social aspects of transitioning can involve a person coming out, changing their name and pronouns, or shifting their gender expression, including clothing, personal grooming like makeup or perfumes and colognes, mannerisms, pitch and tone of voice, and other ways in which we all express gender.

Legal transition

Legal transition involves changing the name and gender marker on legal documents, including driver's licenses, passports, birth certificates, social security cards, insurance information, immigration and naturalization documentation, and many other documents. This is often a very expensive, lengthy, and complicated process.

Having congruent documentation (where the name and gender marker match a person's identity) is important for many reasons. Incongruent documents can out a transgender person, which may put them in a dangerous or vulnerable position. Incongruent documents can cause administrative headaches and lead to denial of important services. For example, insurance companies may reject claims or a person's immigration paperwork may be delayed if the people processing it think there has been a mistake or fraud because the names and gender markers are different on different documents.

There may be times when you are working with a transgender resident and you need to fill out a form with a "sex" designation that does not match the resident's identity, for example, if you are completing paperwork for social security or an insurance claim, certain reimbursements, or other legal documents. If this is the case, the most important thing to do is partner with the resident and make sure they understand that you know and affirm who they are, as well as the limitations and reasons for needing to complete the form a specific way in order for it to be processed. Do not make those decisions for a resident. Instead, partner with them and make it clear you are their advocate. For more information about medical forms and other records see Chapter 3.

Medical transition

Medical transition means using various medical procedures and medications to bring a person's body more in line with their identity. These might include hormone therapies, mastectomy ("top surgery"), breast enhancement, facial feminization surgeries, electrolysis, vaginoplasty or phalloplasty ("bottom surgery") or various other gender affirmation surgeries. These surgeries were previously referred to as "sex reassignment surgeries" but today are more commonly called "gender affirmation surgeries" or "gender-affirming medical procedures."

Transitioning is a process, not an event

Some people may think, incorrectly, that transitioning is a one-time event, or that someone needs to medically transition to "become" a "real" man or woman. It is best to think of transitioning as a process that means something unique to every person, and only that person can say when they feel they have transitioned. Some people may only change their gender expression and never utilize any means of medical transition—a recent survey found that only 25 percent of respondents reported having had some form of transition-related surgery (James et al. 2016). Some people may have no interest in surgery, others may want to have surgery but face barriers to accessing it. Gender affirming medical procedures are often difficult to access and expensive, and many older adults may have health conditions that prevent them from safely having surgery.

There is no one moment when someone transitions; each individual decides if and when they have finished their transition, and it is rude to ask someone about their transition, as these questions are intrusive and personal. If you are a health provider it may be necessary to know details about a resident's medical transition (for example, if they are currently taking hormones), but these questions are only appropriate if you can provide a clear medical or professional reason that you need that information. Otherwise, asking questions about a transgender person's genitals or body, transition, or other personal information is never appropriate.

Some residents may be very open about identifying as transgender or being a person of transgender experience. Others may not identify as transgender, and instead identify only as a man or woman. These people may not wish to ever discuss having been assigned a different sex or their life history, and do not want the fact that they are a person of transgender experience to be known to staff or other residents. Either way, knowing that a person was assigned a sex at birth that is different from how they identify may be important medical information. For example, transgender men may still need cervical cancer screening or pap smears, and transgender women may need prostate exams. This underscores the importance of LGBT-inclusive move-in documents, as discussed in Chapter 3.

Even when discussing a person's history, always use their current and correct name and pronouns, do not switch names or pronouns when talking about their past, and use the phrases "before transitioning" and "after transitioning" rather than "when you were still a man/woman." For example, if Mary is a transgender woman who uses feminine pronouns, always refer to her with she/her pronouns and with the name Mary. If you are discussing her childhood, continue to use she/her pronouns and if you need to discuss a particular point in time you can say, "when you were a child," or "back in 1965," rather than pointing out the time period by discussing her gender. Never use a person's old name. Referring to someone by their old name is often referred to as "deadnaming" and is very hurtful and disrespectful. If you use someone's old name or pronoun by accident, calmly correct yourself, if appropriate, apologize, and move on.

CREATING A POSITIVE COMMUNITY FOR TRANSGENDER RESIDENTS

Check assumptions at the door

We spend all day making assumptions about other people's gender identities based on how they look or sound. Instead of guessing how a person identifies, create opportunities for people to tell you their correct name and the pronouns they use. You can introduce yourself saying, "My name is Tim Johnston—feel free to call me Tim—and I use the pronouns he/him." Making that a habit can invite other people to share how they want to be identified. We all have the right to be addressed the way we want. I hate being called Timothy or Timmy: some residents prefer being addressed as Mr. or Mrs., while others may prefer something more casual. A transgender person may have a different legal name than the name they use in daily life, so it's important to go beyond their paperwork and learn the name they use and stick to it.

If a resident comes out to you as transgender, thank them for telling you and ask if they would like to discuss it further or if they have any specific concerns. Do not comment on their physical appearance, and do not ask questions about their previous name, their personal history, or transitioning. If staff and community members knew someone before they came out and transitioned, at first it may be challenging to remember to use the correct name and pronouns. If you accidently use the incorrect name or pronoun, politely apologize, acknowledge your mistake, and affirm the resident's correct name and pronouns.

When it comes to names and pronouns, practice makes perfect. One of my friends had a cousin who transitioned, and when she came out she asked that everyone to start using the name Ashley, as well as female pronouns. My friend struggled at first, so he started to practice, and while doing the dishes or running he would say things like, "Ashley is my cousin. She is coming over to dinner. We will have her favorite dessert." It may sound silly, but these simple repetitions helped him build new habits so that now he can easily and fluently use his cousin's correct name and pronoun.

BOX 10.1   REVEREND ERIN PROIE'S STORY

A resident came to me very upset because she had just found out her granddaughter was, as she said, in the process of "turning into a boy." This resident was confused by this news, saying things like, "I just don't understand." We spoke about some of the information I had learned during our LGBT training. I asked her to imagine what it must feel like to be uncomfortable in your body, and we talked about the suicide rates in the transgender community. At the end of each visit, we spoke of not needing to fully understand why her grandson was transitioning and also how it was imperative that she make her grandson feel loved. After a few visits, my resident was able to say her grandson's preferred name but still struggled with using masculine pronouns. I affirmed to her that coming out was a sign of trust, again and again keeping her focus on their love. My resident passed away unexpectedly but I believe she was at peace with her grandson's identity, and her grandson knows he was loved by his grandmother.

Reverend Erin Proie, M.Div
Chaplain, United Church Homes

Policies

Over the past several years, politicians have created controversy around transgender people accessing bathrooms, locker rooms, and other sex-segregated spaces. Several laws and policies attempted to force transgender people to use the bathroom associated with the sex they were assigned at birth, rather than the bathroom that matches their identity and expression. This is also a concern in other institutional spaces like schools, prisons, and shelters.

Everyone should be able to access the sex-specific facilities and rooms that match their identity. That is to say, transgender women should be able to use the women's restroom and have a female roommate, and transgender men should be able to use the men's room and have a male roommate. This is an important way to affirm a resident's identity, but crucially it also helps protect them from being harassed or hurt if they are forced to use the wrong restroom, locker room, or other sex-segregated space. In addition to this policy, you can purchase new signs to relabel single-stall bathrooms to be all-gender or gender-neutral bathrooms.

BOX 10.2   CENTERING TRANSGENDER INCLUSION

Some residents, staff, and family members are uncomfortable with the suggestion that everyone, transgender and cisgender people alike, should have access to sex-segregated spaces like bathrooms based on their identity, regardless of if they have had any hormone therapy or surgery. I have met with many administrators and directors who are worried about how residents and families will react.

These conversations are good opportunities to educate staff, families, and residents about the importance of respecting transgender older adults. Here are a few things to remember:

- **Always center the transgender person**: For example, transgender people are at risk of violence or harassment if they are forced to use the wrong bathroom or locker room. Having a clear policy around access based on gender identity is a way to help make everyone safer.

- **Focus on the people, not identities**: A person's transgender identity is private information and should not be revealed to roommates without the transgender resident's permission. If a resident refuses to share a room with a transgender roommate, ask yourself if it is really about the new roommate's transgender identity or if perhaps there is a personality conflict or something else going on. If the conflict persists, it is the roommate refusing to share space with the transgender resident who should be required to move.
- **Build bridges across experience**: If family members are upset about your community's transgender-inclusive policies, have them consider if they would react the same way if a new resident was a different race, ethnicity, or religion. We do not tolerate discrimination based on those identities; why is being transgender any different?
- **A rising tide lifts all boats**: Making your community more inclusive for transgender older adults is not political or special treatment; it reflects your commitment to respecting all people, and everyone will benefit from staff, residents, and families being more diverse and accepting of others. These policies are not "zero-sum," meaning that treating one group with respect does not take anything away from anyone else; it makes the space better for all of us. Remember that even if you do not have transgender residents, visitors or staff may identify as transgender, and creating a more welcoming space will be important for them, as well.

In addition to a community nondiscrimination policy, consider adding explicit language into your resident handbook affirming that each resident has the right to express their gender in whatever way they choose. Make sure that staff, including at salons and barber shops, are aware of this right and feel comfortable helping residents who need help with dressing and grooming. For model language and explanations of why these and other policies are important see the guide "Creating Equal Access to Quality Health Care for Transgender Patients: Transgender-Affirming Hospital Policies" (Lambda Legal et al. 2016), available at hrc.org.

BOX 10.3   SARA DENT'S STORY

Several years ago, I was working as an administrator at a skilled nursing facility, and a transgender woman came to live in our community. At first staff were concerned that other residents would react poorly and it would be difficult to find her a roommate. I connected with the new resident and asked if it was OK for me to disclose her identity in order to find a good match. One of my other female residents volunteered right away, and they got along great! Like with any relationship making a new resident feel welcome is all about communication and trust.

Sara Dent, NHA, MBA
Executive Director
Denver, Colorado

Privacy

At the end of the day, each resident can choose how much they want to reveal about their personal history and identity. Transgender residents may be outed by being asked to remove their clothing, by incongruent documentation, or by staff or other residents. A person's transgender identity should be confidential information, and information about a person's medical transition is confidential medical information protected by HIPAA. Staff should never out a resident without their permission.

BOX 10.4   EXCERPTS FROM THE BOOK *TO SURVIVE ON THIS SHORE*

To Survive on This Shore: Photographs and Interviews with Transgender and Gender Nonconforming Older Adults by Jess T. Dugan and Vanessa Fabbre is a collection of portraits and personal stories centered on the lives of transgender and gender nonconforming older adults. It is a resource for anyone looking to better understand what it means to grow older as a person of transgender experience or a person who is gender nonconforming. Below I have taken three excerpts from the text that address senior living or long-term care:

> My dad has Alzheimer's, which often results in people having long-term memory but remembering nothing in the short term. After I came out to him as transgender, he never got my name wrong, he never messed up my pronouns. He sent me a birthday card that said, "To my son." I remember how that hit me, I went and I cried. You know, it was the kind of acceptance that you hope for but don't expect. But all of a sudden, he wasn't able to recognize who I was. In his memory, he had two daughters. He started telling me stories from his Army days . . . and I started realizing he was connecting with someone else. His best Army buddy was my uncle. So I realized he thought I was him . . . So I'm looking at my dad and I'm thinking, "What happens when I end up in this situation?" I need to get my papers in order. I need to make sure I have end of life stuff written out. Because by the point at which you are no longer able to make those decisions and you begin forgetting things, what if I forget I'm trans? If they are dressing me differently in this place because of my body, then am I gonna know the difference? And who's doing to advocate for me?
>
> —Mitch, 55, Seattle WA

> Now, on the brighter side, this is the best time of my life. I am having an absolute blast . . . I wish I had another fifty years. But I don't want to be one hundred years old if I'm decrepit and need help. It kills me to think that I would go to a nursing home. No frickin' way. I want to stay healthy and die in my bed peacefully. No fanfare, no craziness.
>
> – Barbara, 70, Long Island, NY

> I don't have any concerns about aging, per se, because I don't think our issues are terribly different from anybody else who's aging. I think the greatest fear for me is the greatest fear for anybody who's in a couple, that my partner will pass away. I'm also worried about the lack of nursing homes and long-term care facilities geared toward our community. Right now, if something happened and I needed to be in a home, finding a place where I would be comfortable would be a challenge. I'm hopeful that in twenty years, something will change, preferably sooner rather than later.
>
> – Mike, 55, Palm Springs CA

Learn more about the book at www.tosurviveonthisshore.com

We all have the right to express our gender and be treated with respect. Even if you do not have any transgender residents, you probably will soon, and almost certainly some staff or family members identify as transgender or another gender identity. Creating a more inclusive environment can help everyone feel more comfortable in your community.

SUGGESTIONS

- Always use the correct name and pronouns when referring to everyone. If you accidently use the incorrect name or pronoun, politely apologize, acknowledge your mistake, and affirm the person's correct name and pronouns.
- Remember that everyone has the right to determine how they dress and their personal grooming. If a resident needs help with personal grooming, staff should respect and complete their requests, allowing each resident to choose how they dress and express their gender.
- Many transgender older adults may not identify as transgender, simply referring to themselves as men or women. This should be respected, while also creating a space where they can signal that they are a person of transgender experience in order to receive appropriate medical care.

FURTHER READING AND VIEWING

"Accord Alliance" (www.accordalliance.org/).
"Creating Equal Access to Quality Health Care for Transgender Patients: Transgender-Affirming Hospital Policies" (www.hrc.org/).
To Survive on This Shore: Photographs and Interviews with Transgender and Gender Nonconforming Older Adults by Jess T. Dugan and Vanessa Fabbre.
"Trans Aging: We're Still Here!—Transgender Rights Toolkit: A Legal Guide For Trans People and Their Advocates" (www.lambdalegal.org/).
"Transgender Aging Network (TAN)" (https://forge-forward.org/aging/).

REFERENCES

Accord Alliance. n.d. "Accord Alliance: Frequently Asked Questions." *Accord Alliance*. www.accordalliance.org/learn-about-dsd/faqs/.
Blackless, Melanie, Anthony Charuvastra, Amanda Derryck, Anne Fausto-Sterling, Karl Lauzanne, and Ellen Lee. 2000. "How Sexually Dimorphic Are We? Review and Synthesis." *American Journal of Human Biology* 12 (2): 151–66. https://doi.org/10.1002/(SICI)1520-6300(200003/04)12:2<151::AID-AJHB1>3.0.CO;2-F.
Cook-Daniels, Loree, and michael munson. 2010. "Sexual Violence, Elder Abuse, and Sexuality of Transgender Adults, Age 50+: Results of Three Surveys." *Journal of GLBT Family Studies* 6 (2): 142–77. https://doi.org/10.1080/15504281003705238.
Dugan, Jess T., and Vanessa Fabbre. 2018. *To Survive on This Shore: Photographs and Interviews with Transgender and Gender Nonconforming Older Adults*. Berlin: Kehrer Verlag.
Fredriksen-Goldsen, Karen I., Hyun-Jun Kim, Charles A. Emlet, Anna Muraco, Elena A. Erosheva, Charles P. Hoy-Ellis, Jayn Goldsen, and Heidi Petry. 2011. "The Aging and Health Report: Disparities and Resilience among Lesbian, Gay, Bisexual, and Transgender Older Adults." Seattle, WA: Caring and Aging with Pride. www.age-pride.org/wordpress/wp-content/uploads/2011/05/Full-Report-FINAL-11-16-11.pdf.
Grant, J.M., L. Mottet, J. Tanis, J. Harrison, J.L. Herman, and M. Keisling. 2011. "Injustice at Every Turn: A Report of the National Transgender Discrimination Survey." Washington, D.C.: National Center for Transgender Equality.
James, S.E., J.L. Herman, S. Rankin, M. Keisling, L. Mottet, and M. Anafi. 2016. "The Report of the 2015 U.S. Transgender Survey." Washington, D.C.: National Center for

Transgender Equality. https://transequality.org/sites/default/files/docs/usts/USTS-Full-Report-Dec17.pdf.

Lambda Legal, The Human Rights Campaign, Hogan Lovells, New York City Bar. 2016. "Creating Equal Access to Quality Health Care for Transgender Patients: Transgender-Affirming Hospital Policies." *HRC*. www.hrc.org/resources/transgender-affirming-hospital-policies.

Sax, Leonard. 2002. "How Common Is Intersex? A Response to Anne Fausto-Sterling." *Journal of Sex Research* 39 (3): 174–78. https://doi.org/10.1080/00224490209552139.

11

OLDER ADULTS WITH HIV/AIDS

SUMMARY

In the early 1980s when the first people in the United States were dying from what later became known as AIDS (acquired immunodeficiency syndrome), which is caused by HIV (human immunodeficiency virus), the diagnosis was seen as a death sentence. Today, advances in medical treatments have transformed it into a chronic illness when treated properly, and many more people are growing older and aging well while living with HIV. This chapter describes some general best practices for working with residents with HIV or AIDS, as well as some of the history of the disease and the unique stigma attached to it.

OBJECTIVES

- Learn about the history of HIV/AIDS and how it may impact residents.
- Discuss some of the psychosocial and health disparities faced by people with HIV and long-term survivors.
- Dispel myths about how HIV is transmitted.
- Review privacy protections and ways to combat the stigma faced by people living with HIV/AIDS.

A SHORT HISTORY OF THE HIV/AIDS EPIDEMIC FROM THE 1930s TO TODAY

Scientists believe that the first genetic mutations that would later become HIV happened periodically in Africa sometime in the 1930s. Looking back, several deaths from the 50s to the 70s can be attributed to HIV/AIDS, but it was in 1981 that gay men in Los Angeles and New York started coming down with a rare form of pneumonia called *Pneumocystis carinii* (PCP) or a rare cancer called *Kaposi sarcoma* (KS), which would later be linked to HIV and AIDS. Initially referred to as "GRID" (gay-related immune deficiency syndrome), in 1985 it was given the name "human immunodeficiency virus," or HIV. While we often say HIV/AIDS together, in fact HIV is a virus that, if left untreated, causes AIDS. AIDS is defined as a compromised immune system (CD4 count less than 200 cells/mm3) or by the presence of an opportunistic infection or AIDS-defining condition. People with AIDS have severely compromised immune systems, which makes them susceptible to other diseases like pneumonia.

The United States government was slow to acknowledge the epidemic and only began to act after intense pressure and protests led by activist groups like AIDS Coalition to Unleash Power (ACT UP) and the Gay Men's Health Crisis (GMHC). During this time, many people with HIV were treated very poorly by medical providers, often denied treatment or kept in quarantine units, with providers unwilling to interact with them or, in some cases, touch them or enter their rooms to remove bedpans or food. As awareness of the disease widened, but without concrete knowledge about risk factors or an explanation for how the virus was transmitted, there was an intense homophobic and anti-HIV/AIDS backlash. The combination of stigmatization and the government's disregard for people suffering during the epidemic made many people who lived through that time deeply distrusting of the government, health care providers, and other large institutions, which were seen as indifferent at best, hostile at worst. Even today, some providers are unaware of how HIV is transmitted or may not have completely accurate information. As I will discuss later on, HIV cannot be transmitted through casual contact, so the precautions medical care providers should take when working with a resident living with HIV are primarily to make sure that the care provider does not transmit an infection to the person living with HIV/AIDS, who may have a weaker immune system.

Because of this history, many people associate the HIV/AIDS epidemic in the United States with men who have sex with men, but today many people with HIV are heterosexual or may not identify as members of the LGBT community. This is particularly true when we extend our view beyond the United States. The disease has had a much wider impact in other countries, and that impact intersects with the history of colonialism and global inequality. During the late 1980s and the 1990s, HIV spread across Africa. By 1986, 5–10 percent of people in Zaire, Rwanda, Uganda, Kenya, Zambia, and Central African Republic were HIV positive, roughly 10 to 20 times the rate in the United States (Engel 2006). Today, approximately 36.9 million people worldwide are living with HIV/AIDS, and the populations with the highest risk of contracting HIV are men who have sex with men, injection drug users, female sex workers, and transgender women (UNAIDS 2018). Of the 36.9 million people with HIV, 2.2 million live in Western and Central Europe and North America, while the highest number of people living with HIV/AIDS are in Eastern and Southern Africa (19.6 million), Western and Central Africa (6.1 million), and Asia and the Pacific (5.2 million) (UNAIDS 2018).

Today in the United States, the number of new diagnoses has remained stable overall, but Black/African-American and Hispanic/Latino men who have sex with men are disproportionally represented (CDC 2018c). Of the transgender people diagnosed between 2009–14, over 80 percent were transgender women, over half were Black/African-American, and almost half lived in the South (CDC 2018b). These high rates are often the result of poverty, lack of access to healthcare, and a lack of harm reduction programs for people using substances.

HIV/AIDS AND AGING

Advances in treatment mean that today HIV is a chronic illness, and with proper treatment a person can have a low enough viral load that the disease does not progress to AIDS or does so much more slowly. Because people with HIV are living long lives, by 2015, 47 percent of Americans living with HIV were over the age of 50 (CDC 2018a).

People who have been living with HIV for many years—especially those diagnosed before 1995, when effective treatments were developed—are often referred to as "long-term survivors." Many long-term survivors assumed their diagnosis meant they would be dead within a year or two, so they spent all of their money or did not make investments in retirement funds or long-term care insurance. As a result, they may be more economically vulnerable today. Others experience "survivor's guilt," questioning why they are still alive when their loved ones are not, and have complicated feelings of grief, guilt, and relief.

As discussed in Chapter 8, our society de-sexualizes older adults, and many people do not consider the fact that residents may be living with HIV or may become newly infected through sexual activity or drug use. Some older adults may not use preventative measures or barriers during sex, which can lead to an increase in sexually transmitted infections, including HIV. It is also the case that older adults are rarely tested and diagnosed, either because their providers do not know they are sexually active or using injectable drugs or because they are misdiagnosed due to the fact that the signs and symptoms of HIV resemble other age-related and chronic illnesses. Once a person has received a diagnosis, their HIV status is medical information protected by HIPAA, and it is the resident's decision whether they want to disclose their HIV status to staff or other residents. Organizations like SAGE advocate for routine testing at any age, as well as making preventative supplies and education available to all older adults in senior residential settings. One simple way to encourage safer sex is to make external and internal condoms and dental dams available for free to all residents.

Some people think that an HIV diagnosis is the end of someone's sex life—but that is not true. With proper treatment and adherence to medication regimens, the HIV viral load can be kept so low that it is undetectable and extremely unlikely to be transmitted to another person (CDC 2018d). People with HIV have the right to be sexually active; it is important that all parties can make informed decisions and have access to barriers such as condoms. Medication adherence is crucial to maintain a low viral load and decrease the probability of transmission between sexual partners.

A relatively new advance is a class of drugs known as pre-exposure prophylaxis, or PrEP. PrEP can be taken daily and can greatly reduce the likelihood of transmitting HIV through sexual activity. PrEP does not prevent the transmission of any other sexually transmitted infections, and people using PrEP are encouraged to still use condoms and other barriers.

Finally, people with HIV may experience what is called "HIV-associated dementia" or "AIDS Dementia Complex" (ADC). The symptoms are similar to other dementias, but unlike Alzheimer's, which is irreversible and has no cure, some symptoms of ADC can be treated or improved through the use of antiretroviral therapies. ADC is not common, and many older people with HIV may notice other changes to cognitive function that are caused by things like a history of substance use or other medications. Many of the same dementia care recommendations in Chapter 12 apply here, and staff should take into account the resident's experience of living through the HIV epidemic, as well as the stigma associated with the disease, when considering how to create the resident's dementia care plan. For example, people with HIV may also experience depression or post-traumatic stress disorder, both of which can influence behavior and agitation or impact cognitive functioning and must be addressed in the care plan.

People with HIV face stigmas that can have a negative impact on their health and make them more likely to face isolation (Brennan-Ing 2018). People living with HIV are also more likely to have multiple chronic conditions or multimorbidities that require treatment and are at a higher risk for polypharmacy (Sangarlangkarn and Appelbaum 2016). Depression is one of the most common comorbidities. People living with HIV have rates of depression five times greater than noninfected adults (Brennan-Ing 2016), and studies have shown a relationship between depression and medication nonadherence (Gonzalez et al. 2011). Staff should be on the lookout for signs of psychological distress and consider ways to keep residents living with HIV integrated into the community, in charge of their own health, and constantly developing and reinforcing multiple coping strategies (Rueda, Law, and Rourke 2014). Similar to LGBT people who have lived through difficult times, people living with HIV have survived intense stigmas and often draw from those reservoirs of strength and support to confront the challenges faced by aging as a person with HIV.

BOX 11.1   LIVING AND AGING PROUDLY WITH HIV IN A LONG-TERM CARE HOME

With the arrival of antiretroviral therapy, HIV has transformed into a manageable illness, but the social stigma, discrimination, rejection, and shame of HIV continue. A large percentage of people living with HIV infections are gay men and also transgender women. As gay men and trans women age, the decision to live in a long-term care home is a frightening reality. Some of them chose to go into the closet and others are confronted with the complex issues of what and when to disclose. Do they disclose their sexual orientation, gender identity, HIV status or all of them? How will care providers and other residents react?

We explore the success story of a man living at Rekai Centres, a senior residence in Toronto. The resident is over 70 but has a youthful demeanor and a bubbly personality. He has mild dementia and he was diagnosed HIV positive in the 1990s. He has lived at the Rekai Centres in Toronto for many years.

He is outspoken and very candid about his life in his youth, his sexual orientation, HIV status, supportive biological family, friends, and artwork. His room is filled with memorabilia of his life; photographs of his gay friends, his parents, brother, sisters, and nieces and nephews, along with rainbow signs, news clipping of historical events, and the products of his passion for the visual arts. In his senior years he has said he wanted to live openly as a gay man and not hide his identity or his HIV status. He is still surprised he has lived this long with HIV with robust health. The open environment and inclusive, person-centered care at Rekai Centres reduces isolation and loneliness and improves mental and emotional health for the residents.

This philosophy is further echoed by Barbara Mihalik, Director of Community Partnerships, Programs and Volunteer Services at Rekai Centres. She strongly emphasizes the need to provide services with a heart and soul and with a person-centered focus and dedication to equity for sexual and gender minorities. She stresses "the importance of gearing services towards the residents, the comfort zone of the resident, how you define culture and where the residents are most comfortable." Rekai Centres has policies and a code of conduct, and training is offered to staff at the center for sensitivity and cultural competency. The in-house intake forms provide residents the options to self-identity their sexual orientation, gender, and gender pronouns. The board at Rekai Centres is supportive of the equity work for LGBT2SQ (lesbian, gay, bisexual, transgender, two-spirit, queer) seniors and the inclusive, respectful, welcoming environment for all residents of all intersectional identities, cultures, ethnicities, and races.

Devan Nambiar, MSc. has been working in the HIV and LGBT2SQ sector for over 20 years and provides training and education to health care and social services providers. For more information, www.ghis.ca.

Learn more by reading the *LGBT Tool Kit: Creating Lesbian, Gay, Bisexual, Trans Inclusive and Affirming Care and Services* by Toronto Long-Term Care Homes and Services, 2017, available at www.rainbowhealthontario.ca.

Devan Nambiar

STIGMAS AND MYTHS ABOUT HIV/AIDS

Staff or residents may be uncomfortable interacting with people who are open about being HIV positive. This discomfort reflects the strong stigma associated with HIV, much of which is rooted in the anti-LGBT history of the epidemic, or the incorrect judgement that people get HIV/AIDS because they are promiscuous, careless, or drug users. It is important for staff to recognize and work to move past these stigmas and moral judgements if they are going to treat each resident with respect.

Others may not make judgements about residents living with HIV, but fear them because they do not understand what HIV/AIDS is or how HIV is transmitted from one person to another. HIV is transmitted through some bodily fluids, including blood, semen, pre-seminal fluids, rectal fluids, vaginal fluids, and breast milk. It cannot be transmitted through saliva, sneezing, coughing, sharing bathrooms, bathing, or other casual contact. Most transmissions in the United States occur through sexual activity or sharing injection drug equipment (HHS 2018). Casual contact is completely safe, and there is no reason for staff or residents to behave any differently when sharing space with a resident who is HIV positive. Nursing staff who administer insulin or other injections should follow regular precautions for the transmission of blood-borne infections (CDC 2007).

In general, the normal precautions staff take to avoid exchanging bodily fluids with residents, such as wearing gloves or face masks, are sufficient to prevent the transmission of HIV. In fact, while it is true that these precautions can protect staff, they are intended to stop staff from transmitting their infections to people with HIV. People with HIV have weakened immune systems, and staff need to make sure that they do what they can to help the resident avoid getting sick.

A resident's HIV/AIDS status is medical information and is protected by HIPAA. If staff or other residents are gossiping about a resident's HIV/AIDS status they are violating the resident's privacy and creating a potentially hostile or harmful environment for the resident.

Older adults living with HIV/AIDS, whether they are long-term survivors or newly diagnosed, face unique social and medical challenges, and they deserve the same respectful, high-quality treatment as everyone else in your community. Breaking through the stigma and giving staff accurate information can help them see that they already have the skills they need to provide excellent and equitable care to people with HIV. Training can capitalize on this existing expertise, and open, fact-based conversations about HIV and AIDS in the older adult demographic are an essential way to ensure everyone in your community can meet the needs of this population and dispel any myths or fears they may have about working with people living with HIV/AIDS.

Organizations like ACRIA (acria.org/training-center), SAGE (sageusa.org), and the National Network of STD Clinical Prevention Training Centers (nnptc.org), can provide training and education resources, and many federally qualified health centers and local LGBT community centers or HIV/AIDS organizations provide testing, counseling, and other resources in your local community.

SUGGESTIONS

- Remember that safety protocols are primarily for ensuring that the care provider does not transmit an infection to the person living with HIV/AIDS.
- A person's HIV/AIDS status is private medical information protected by HIPAA.
- Ensure that residents have access to condoms and barriers, as well as information on sexual health from trustworthy and accurate sources.
- Educate staff on HIV and AIDS, including common misinformation, myths, and best practices to protect their health and that of the resident.

FURTHER READING AND VIEWING

"Age Is Not a Condom" (http://ageisnotacondom.org/en/home/).
"Aging Pozitively" (www.lgbtagingcenter.org/resources/resource.cfm?r=313).
"Eight Policy Recommendations for Improving the Health and Wellness of Older Adults with HIV—Diverse Elders Coalition" (www.diverseelders.org).
"A Greying Pandemic" (http://agrayingpandemic.org/).
"United in Anger: A History of ACT UP" (www.unitedinanger.com/).
We Were Here (film) (https://wewereherefilm.com/).

REFERENCES

Brennan-Ing, Mark. 2016. "HIV/AIDS and Aging." In *The SAGE Encyclopedia of LGBTQ Studies*, edited by Abbie E. Goldberg. 2455 Teller Road, Thousand Oaks, California 91320: SAGE Publications, Inc. https://doi.org/10.4135/9781483371283.n189.

———. 2018. "Diversity, Stigma, and Social Integration among Older Adults with HIV." *European Geriatric Medicine*, December. https://doi.org/10.1007/s41999-018-0142-3.

CDC. 2007. "Guideline for Isolation Precautions: Preventing Transmission of Infectious Agents in Healthcare Settings." *Centers for Disease Control and Prevention*. https://www.cdc.gov/infectioncontrol/guidelines/isolation/index.html.

———. 2018a. "Diagnoses of HIV Infection among Adults Aged 50 Years and Older in the United States and Dependent Areas, 2011–2016." *HIV Surveillance Supplemental Report* 23 (5). www.cdc.gov/hiv/pdf/library/reports/surveillance/cdc-hiv-surveillance-supplemental-report-vol-23-5.pdf.

———. 2018b. "HIV and Transgender People." *Centers for Disease Control and Prevention*. https://www.cdc.gov/hiv/pdf/group/gender/transgender/cdc-hiv-transgender-factsheet.pdf.

———. 2018c. "HIV in the United States." *Centers for Disease Control and Prevention*. December 7, 2018. https://www.cdc.gov/hiv/statistics/overview/ataglance.html.

———. 2018d. "HIV Treatment as Prevention." *Centers for Disease Control and Prevention*. December 18, 2018. https://www.cdc.gov/hiv/risk/art/index.html.

Engel, Jonathan. 2006. *The Epidemic: A Global History of AIDS*. New York: Smithsonian Books/Collins.

Gonzalez, Jeffrey S., Abigail W. Batchelder, Christina Psaros, and Steven A. Safren. 2011. "Depression and HIV/AIDS Treatment Nonadherence: A Review and Meta-Analysis." *JAIDS: Journal of Acquired Immune Deficiency Syndromes* 58 (2): 181–87. https://doi.org/10.1097/QAI.0B013E31822D490A.

HHS. 2018. "The Basics of HIV Prevention." *U.S. Department of Health and Human Services*. October 2018. https://aidsinfo.nih.gov/understanding-hiv-aids/fact-sheets/20/48/the-basics-of-hiv-prevention.

Rueda, Sergio, Stephanie Law, and Sean B. Rourke. 2014. "Psychosocial, Mental Health, and Behavioral Issues of Aging with HIV." *Current Opinion in HIV and AIDS* 9 (4): 325–31. https://doi.org/10.1097/COH.0000000000000071.

Sangarlangkarn, Aroonsiri, and Jonathan S. Appelbaum. 2016. "Caring for Older Adults with the Human Immunodeficiency Virus." *Journal of the American Geriatrics Society* 64 (11): 2322–29. https://doi.org/10.1111/jgs.14584.

UNAIDS. 2018. "Fact Sheet—World AIDS Day 2018." *UNAIDS*. www.unaids.org/sites/default/files/media_asset/UNAIDS_FactSheet_en.pdf.

12

DEMENTIA, MEMORY CARE, AND LGBT PEOPLE

SUMMARY

Alzheimer's disease and other dementias present unique challenges for LGBT older adults, including family dynamics, sexual expression, and gender identity and expression. This chapter outlines what makes LGBT people with dementia unique, the challenges facing LGBT caregivers of any older adult living with dementia, and some specific considerations for staff working in a memory care setting.

OBJECTIVES

- Understand how the dementia disease process and associated behavioral changes may be treated differently or unfairly in the case of LGBT older adults than in the non-LGBT population.
- Examine ways to create environments that send a message of inclusion and safety.
- Learn how to use advanced directives to preserve and advocate for an LGBT older adult's wishes as they become less able to articulate their desires.

ALZHEIMER'S DISEASE AND OTHER DEMENTIAS

According to the Alzheimer's Association, one in three older adults will die with Alzheimer's disease or another form of dementia (Alzheimer's Association 2018). These other forms can include dementia related to a traumatic brain injury, vascular dementia, Lewy Body dementia, dementia caused by HIV/AIDS, or dementia symptoms that are a part of another disease. In this chapter, I use "dementia" as an umbrella term for decreased executive functioning, decreased ability to recall and create memories, impaired reasoning, lessened impulse control, and personality changes.

There are currently 5.7 million people living with Alzheimer's disease, and that number could rise as high as 14 million by the year 2050 (Alzheimer's Association 2018). This intersects with the growing number of LGBT older adults, meaning that memory care communities and other dementia care providers are likely going to see an increase in the number of LGBT people accessing their services. Race and ethnicity are also factors: African-Americans are around twice as likely to have Alzheimer's disease and Hispanic older adults are about one and a half times more likely to have the disease than white older adults (Alzheimer's Association 2018). Asian-Americans and Pacific Islanders (AAPI) are one of the fastest growing groups of older adults in the United States, and over half of AAPI older adults have limited English language proficiency, making linguistic cultural competency doubly important to both diagnose dementia and support AAPI older adults living with dementia (National Asian Pacific Center on Aging 2013). In addition, LGBT older adults, especially older adults of color, may be more likely to be living with chronic health conditions like diabetes, depression, and high blood pressure, which complicate and may increase the risk of dementia (SAGE 2013). Some of the 5.7 million people living with Alzheimer's who are not LGBT are being cared for by an LGBT family member or friend.

A new report by SAGE and the Alzheimer's Association outlines key areas where LGBT people face additional challenges to navigating living with dementia, including stigma, social isolation, poverty, health disparities, sexuality and gender expression, utilization of aging network services, and living with HIV/AIDS (SAGE and Alzheimer's Association 2018).

Many people sense that they are beginning to become more confused or forgetful but refuse to see a doctor or get tested, often waiting until there is an emergency or they can no longer safely live alone. It is often when these emergencies occur that friends and family learn how bad it has gotten and try to intervene. Hiding these challenges is often rooted in fear, and many people enter into a state of denial when they notice their memory and attention failing.

In addition to fear, there is a lot of stigma around dementia diagnoses. Ageism is just as present in the LGBT community as it is in our wider culture, and I have heard from LGBT people with dementia who feel that they are no longer welcome in LGBT spaces. Sometimes members of their chosen family and friends will pull away, saying that they "don't want to see them like that."

There are other reasons that LGBT people may have trouble accessing the kinds of services that can support them as they navigate dementia. For example, high-quality dementia care is expensive, and a lifetime of employment discrimination has made it difficult for many LGBT older adults, especially transgender older adults and LGBT people of color, to save money or purchase long-term care insurance. Given that so many older people live with some form of dementia, this chapter is intended to help staff provide supportive care to LGBT people with dementia, as well as to LGBT caregivers.

CREATING A SAFER ENVIRONMENT

People living with dementia can be confused about what year it is, where they are, or the identities of people around them. As the disease progresses they usually move backwards in time and have a clearer grasp of memories and emotions from earlier in life. Activities and conversations that focus on reminiscing about memories from the distant past can therefore be soothing and engaging (Alzheimer's Association 2019).

What if you felt comfortable being out of the closet in 2019, but now you think it's 1965? What if you can't remember whether you came out to your nurse, or are confused because staff are using the wrong pronoun to address you? What if you can't tell if the person visiting you is a friend, lover, or stranger? These are just some of the worries that may confront an LGBT person living with dementia. Given that the resident's sense of time, place, and safety will shift as they grow older, there are a number of things staff can do to try to signal that an LGBT person is safe.

Memory care staff are accustomed to controlling the community environment to make sure it is not too noisy, crowded, or stimulating and that there are strong way-finding and context clues such as labels and clear pathways from bedrooms to common areas. The same idea can be applied to communicating LGBT inclusion. Rainbow flags and stickers, images of LGBT people, and inclusive statements can all help ease anxieties. Consider having an openly-LGBT resident write a note to themselves stating that they are safe and can be out to staff. If a resident cannot remember if they are out or if they are safe, reading the note in their own handwriting can help ease their anxieties. Repetition and persistent and permanent symbols of inclusion are key to creating a safer atmosphere.

Staff working with people with dementia benefit from knowing a lot of information about each resident's personal history and their likes, dislikes, hopes, and fears. To that end, Chapter 3 has some suggestions for inclusive intake questions and making the move-in process more LGBT affirming.

Personal history and preferences worksheets allow older adults to communicate important information about their life experiences, which can be helpful for providers as the disease progresses. Likewise, tools like the PELI (Preferences for Everyday Living Inventory) can help capture information about what time the person typically wakes up, when they prefer to shower, how they want to dress and be groomed, their interests and activities, and other information that can help staff provide person-directed care.

These tools can be made more LGBT-inclusive by including prompts like

The pronouns I use are:
Please address me using the name:
The people closest to me are:
Important things you should know about me:

For more information and an example of one such document, see the Rainbow PELI available at www.PreferenceBasedLiving.com. I discussed the Rainbow PELI in more detail in Chapter 3.

When working through these documents the resident may not feel comfortable divulging personal information to staff, so make it clear that they can edit the documents whenever they want, or let residents complete them alone on their own time.

The resident may not feel comfortable discussing their LGBT identity in this initial meeting, so having open conversations free of assumptions can help staff learn about their preferences, personal history, and how they want to be treated as the disease progresses. It may be the case that the resident never affirmatively declares that they are LGBT, but staff can still learn about their history and support network in a way that will be helpful later on.

SHIFTING BEHAVIORS AND IDENTITIES

People living with dementia may do things that to others seem strange and disruptive. As the disease progresses many residents lose impulse control, become much less inhibited, and may start exhibiting new and surprising behaviors. With creative thinking many of these challenging behaviors can be stopped, decreased, or redirected to a private setting where they can be expressed appropriately.

You may be familiar with scenarios like a married woman starting to date a male resident because she cannot remember she has a husband. This can be painful for the family, and supporting the family requires explaining facts about dementia and what kinds of behaviors to expect, and emphasizing that their loved one is not trying to hurt anyone and that she has the right to live her life fully—including having intimate relationships in the community. This woman deserves to be affirmed as the person she is in the present—a person with desires—rather than expecting her to remain who she was before the disease. This same level of care should be extended to LGBT residents or residents behaving in a way consistent with LGBT identities (such as engaging in same-sex sexual contact). In short, it does not matter if the female resident has a boyfriend or a girlfriend; she has the same rights in either case.

One concern raised by advocates for LGBT people with dementia is that their behaviors may be judged more harshly, or that they may face unequitable treatment in how staff respond. In the scenario in the previous paragraph staff may be able to help the family understand the woman's new romance with a male resident but may not know how to react if the woman began a relationship with another woman. Anecdotally, I have heard of staff who see two men or two women becoming affectionate and assume that they are confused or that one person is taking advantage of the other. Staff might make that assumption because they have never considered that the resident may have same-sex attractions and that this new behavior is expressing a genuine desire. If the sexual expression makes staff or family members uncomfortable, they might try to separate the people involved, discourage the relationship, or otherwise prevent the residents from expressing their sexuality. People with dementia deserve privacy, and family members only need to be notified if the behavior presents a safety risk or if there is a need to discuss it in relation to care planning.

It is beyond the scope of this book to outline all the safeguards and best practices staff can use to gauge a resident's ability to consent to sexual contact. Sexual expression and intimacy are important at all ages, and people with dementia can still consent to sexual contact. For more information see the discussion and resources in Chapter 8.

Another common concern is that transgender older adults will lose control over how they are dressed or their gender identity and expression, or will be addressed with the wrong name and pronouns. For example, a transgender man who prefers to dress in pants and be addressed by his masculine name may have family members who deny his identity, use female pronouns, and attempt to prevent staff from dressing him in masculine clothing. This is very serious, and if the resident's identity is not respected it can lead to distress, depression, withdrawal, or other negative outcomes.

Similarly, once when I was training memory care staff a person asked, "We have a male resident who asks to wear dresses one day, and then pants and a button shirt the next. Does this mean he is transgender, and how should staff respond?" It can be easy to make assumptions about this person. Perhaps the resident has always wanted to express a feminine gender identity, and now that the dementia is removing inhibitions they are doing so. However, it could also be an issue of comfort or personal taste and not be connected to the resident's gender identity at all. Unless the resident can articulate a reason behind their behavior, we cannot know the cause. But importantly, we do not need to know the cause in order to treat that resident with respect and care. It is not our job to make decisions for residents, but rather to attend to their verbal and nonverbal communication and provide the environment and supports that allow them to make as many decisions as possible for as long as possible.

In both of these scenarios—the transgender man and the person switching between masculine and feminine clothing—staff can respond by dressing the resident in whatever way that person wants to be dressed. If they ask staff to use a new pronoun or name, take note and respect that request. The key is responding to the person as they are in that moment in time and staying flexible enough to change as they change. If family members struggle with this, encourage them to reach out to PFLAG or other support groups for families of LGBT people.

All of this requires enormous sensitivity, but as we discussed in Chapter 7 no matter how strongly family members may react, the interests and desires of the resident need to be given priority. This is another reason why an LGBT-inclusive and robust intake process is essential. The information gleaned from it can equip staff to advocate for residents even if it requires pushing back against the wishes of family members.

SUPPORTING LGBT CAREGIVERS AND FAMILY MEMBERS

Supporting LGBT caregivers—that is, LGBT people in a caregiving role for family members or friends experiencing dementia—could easily be a whole separate book. What I want to focus on here are some of the unique stresses that LGBT family members of people living with dementia may encounter.

LGBT caregivers may feel less welcome bringing their families, partners, or friends into the caregiving process. Perhaps their parent does not know or accept that they are LGBT or the caregiver fears that providers will discriminate against them. Caregiving is emotionally and at times physically taxing, and if caregivers do not feel like they can lean on their partners or community supports they will experience a higher risk of fatigue and burnout. Asking a caregiver open ended questions like, "Do you have anyone you can talk to when you feel exhausted?" or, "Is there anyone else who can give you a break so you can get some exercise?" can help identify their support network, and the people in that network can be activated to provide support and respite for the primary caregiver.

It might also be the case that a parent doesn't remember that their child is LGBT or is confused about the caregiver's life. Perhaps they keep mistaking the same-sex partner for a friend, or cannot remember that their child has transitioned—they might repeatedly ask for their son, not recognizing her as their daughter. These errors are probably not intentional, but they can still be hurtful. Staff can help ease the pain by explaining the dementia disease process and strategizing with the caregiver about how they want to respond when their parent is confused or agitated. The key is to make sure that LGBT caregivers are given choices about how to respond, and that staff support those decisions as a part of their partnership. One couple might not mind being introduced as friends or a transgender child could be OK introducing herself as a volunteer when her parent doesn't recognize her, but other caregivers might find those adjustments and strategies hurtful. Each caregiver is unique, so training staff on how to have these difficult but important conversations is another example of how an LGBT-inclusive organization not only benefits LGBT residents, but can also help family members and caregivers who identify as LGBT.

ADVANCED DIRECTIVES AND FAMILIES OF CHOICE

As we discussed in Chapter 7, many LGBT older adults rely on chosen families or families of choice. This is particularly important to remember when someone is diagnosed with dementia or showing signs of memory loss, because those chosen family members may not be legally empowered to make decisions for the resident. The same is true for partners who are not married or in a civil union and lack power of attorney. Without such protections a person's biological or legal family members are empowered to make important decisions and can even keep LGBT older adults away from their partners or families of choice.

There are a number of tools that staff can use to help protect LGBT people living with dementia.

The first is to use open-ended questions—e.g. "Tell me about the most important people in your life"—to figure out who the resident's support network and trusted friends are. The resident may not understand that if they become incapacitated, their legal family members will be contacted to make decisions about their care and finances. By asking open-ended questions, staff can begin to see who the people closest to the resident are and empower the resident to choose who they want to grant the legal power to participate in their care. Additionally, a resident's friend, roommate, or partner might need to set up protections to ensure that they are able to remain living in their home, inherit any money or property that the resident wants to pass on to them after they die, and access survivor benefits.

Encouraging residents to complete these advanced directives early on will protect their interests. Certain directives can be edited and used to explicitly outline how a person wants to be treated in the late stages of the disease and after their death, including instructions about names, pronouns, clothing, and visitation. Forms like the Disposition of Bodily Remains can be changed by lawyers to allow the person to say who will be responsible for their funeral arrangements, how they want to be dressed for their funeral, who should be invited (and not invited), and the name to be used in the memorial service and on grave markers (Prachniak 2014). This is particularly important for transgender people who fear their biological or legal family members will not respect their identities or their wishes after they die.

IT TAKES A VILLAGE, AND GREAT COMMUNICATION

I know I sound like a broken record, but each resident is unique, and they will experience dementia in a unique way. When we see residents behaving in a way consistent with LGBT identities it can be tempting to label them as LGBT and make assumptions about their identity. Those assumptions may be inaccurate, and terms LGBT people use might not be meaningful to the resident. What is most important is helping them express autonomy and self-determination for as long as possible. Helping LGBT older adults thrive requires that staff be open, flexible, and willing to navigate the tensions that may arise between residents, biological and chosen families, and others in the community.

SUGGESTIONS

- Do not assume that changes in behavior, especially sexual interest and gender expression or identity, are caused by the dementia. Work collaboratively to identify and then support aspects of the resident's identity or sexual desire that may be being expressed for the first time.
- Do not "out" residents to family members unless it is necessary for their safety, the safety of another resident, or a necessary part of their care plan.
- Train staff to be flexible with terminology, names, and pronouns, as well as to demonstrate patience with residents who may not remember coming out and may do so repeatedly.
- Keep your focus on supporting the resident to be as autonomous and independent as possible, for as long as possible. It is the resident, not staff or family, who decides things like how they are dressed, who can visit, and how they spend their time.

FURTHER READING AND VIEWING

"Issues Brief: LGBT and Dementia" (www.sageusa.org/).
Lesbian, Gay, Bisexual and Trans* Individuals Living with Dementia: Concepts, Practice and Rights by Sue Westwood and Elizabeth Price Editors.
"My Preferences for Everyday Living Inventory (PELI): Rainbow PELI Explainer Sheet" (www. abramsoncenter.org/media/1200/peli-nh-full.pdf).

REFERENCES

Alzheimer's Association. 2018. "2018 Alzheimer's Disease Facts and Figures." *Alzheimer's Association*. www.alz.org/media/HomeOffice/Facts%20and%20Figures/facts-and-figures.pdf.
———. 2019. "Stages and Behaviors." 2019. *Alzheimer's Association* (blog). www.alz.org/help-support/caregiving/stages-behaviors.
National Asian Pacific Center on Aging. 2013. "Asian Americans and Pacific Islanders in the United States Aged 65 Years and Older: Population, Nativity, and Language." *National Asian Pacific Center on Aging Data Brief* 1 (3). www.napca.org/wp-content/uploads/2017/10/65-population-report-FINAL.pdf.
Prachniak, Corey. 2014. "Creating End-of-Life Documents for Trans Individuals: An Advocate's Guide." *The National Resource Center on LGBT Aging and Whitman-Walker Health*. www.lgbtagingcenter.org/resources/resource.cfm?r=694.
SAGE. 2013. "Health Equity and LGBT Older Adults of Color." *SAGE*. www.sageusa.org/resource-posts/health-equity-and-lgbt-elders-of-color-recommendations-for-policy-and-practice/.
SAGE and the Alzheimer's Association. "Issues Brief: LGBT and Dementia." 2018. *SAGE*. www.sageusa.org/wp-content/uploads/2018/08/lgbt-dementia-issues-brief.pdf.

13

RIGHTS AND PROTECTIONS

SUMMARY

There are several state and federal laws and regulations that can protect LGBT older adults from harm and discrimination in senior living settings, as well as ensuring their privacy. This chapter outlines these protections, some troubling trends activists worry may impact LGBT older adults in the coming years, and key considerations for maintaining an LGBT person's privacy while also making sure staff have the information they need to provide person-centered care.

OBJECTIVES

- Understand the federal protections that apply to LGBT older adults and learn how to research state and local protections.
- Consider when it is and is not acceptable to tell another person about a resident's LGBT identity and how to keep that information as private and protected as possible.
- Determine how best to share important information about a person's identity to improve care without outing them or breaking their confidence.

LEGAL PROTECTIONS FOR LGBT OLDER ADULTS

Legal protections for LGBT people of all ages are a patchwork of municipal, state, and federal laws, along with various regulations, policies, and court decisions. This is a constantly changing landscape, and the information in this chapter may soon be out of date. I am assuming that you and your staff know which regulations apply to your particular community; this chapter is intended to show some areas of the law and regulations that may apply to your LGBT residents. I am focusing on three areas: housing and employment discrimination, regulatory compliance, and privacy. This is not comprehensive, and I am not a lawyer, so the information in this chapter should not be understood as legal advice. If you think you or one of your residents has experienced discrimination you should contact a lawyer, legal aid organization (such as Lambda Legal, www.lambdalegal.org/helpdesk or [212] 809–8585), as soon as possible

HOUSING AND EMPLOYMENT DISCRIMINATION

There is no explicit federal legislation to provide blanket basic legal protections for LGBT people. A proposed piece of legislation called the Equality Act would amend the Civil Rights Act of 1964 and several other pieces of federal legislation to include sexual orientation and gender identity as explicitly protected categories, adding them to nondiscrimination laws applied to employment, housing, credit, education, public spaces and services, federally funded programs, and jury service.

Senators Michael Bennet (D-CO), Lisa Murkowski (R-AK), and Bob Casey (D-PA) have introduced a bill at the federal level—the Inclusive Aging Act—which would, among other things, designate LGBT older adults as a group of greatest social need within the Older Americans Act. Representative Suzanne Bonamici (D-OR1) has introduced the Ruthie and Connie LGBT Elder Americans Act in the House, and both she and Representative Debra Haaland (D-NM1) have introduced the Elder Pride Act. Together, those bills mirror the Senate's Inclusive Aging Act.

Currently none of these pieces of federal legislation have passed.

In terms of low-income or affordable housing, the HUD Equal Access Rules are a set of three rules, the first of which extends protections to people based on their actual or perceived sexual orientation, gender identity, or marital status across housing that is assisted by HUD or financed by a mortgage insured by the Federal Housing Authority. The second rule instructs core shelter programs to provide access to single-sex shelters and services in accordance with a person's gender identity, and the third rule extends the protections in the first rule to include HUD's Native American and Native Hawaiian programs.

The HUD LGBTQ Resources Page summarizes LGBTQ rights as follows:

Know Your Rights under the Fair Housing Act and HUD's Rules:

- It is prohibited under the Fair Housing Act for any landlord or housing provider to discriminate against LGBTQ persons because of their real or perceived gender identity or any other reason that constitutes sex based discrimination.
- It is illegal for any landlord or housing provider to deny housing because of someone's HIV/AIDS status under the Fair Housing Act and the Americans with Disabilities Act.
- It is prohibited for a lender to deny an FHA-insured mortgage to any qualified applicant based on their sexual orientation, gender identity, or marital status.
- It is prohibited for any landlord or housing provider who receives HUD or FHA funds to discriminate against a tenant on the basis of real or perceived sexual orientation, gender identity or marital status.
- It is prohibited for all homeless facilities to segregate or isolate transgender individuals solely based on their gender identity.

(HUD n.d.)

Senior living communities that accept HUD vouchers or make use of HUD financing must abide by the Equal Access Rules. Complaints can be filed by contacting HUD's Office of Fair Housing and Equal Opportunity at (800) 669–9777 or contacting another legal aid organization.

Several states have enacted legislation and regulations intended to protect LGBT elders, including California, Massachusetts, and Illinois. Many other states and municipalities have housing and employment nondiscrimination laws that protect LGBT people, including LGBT older adults. The Movement Advancement Project (www.lgbtmap.org/) has resources to help you determine which protections apply in your state.

LICENSING AND REGULATORY COMPLIANCE

Recent Centers for Medicare and Medicaid Services (CMS) survey regulations do not contain explicit guidance or requirements to train staff on LGBT cultural competency, but they do require that new nursing home residents be given care plans that accord with the goals of person-centered care, including "incorporat[ing] the resident's personal and cultural preferences in developing goals of care" (CMS 2017). Taking into account a resident's personal and cultural preferences requires that staff are trained to ask open-ended questions, create an environment where LGBT residents feel comfortable being honest about their personal and cultural preferences, and that staff have the skills they need to meet those requests. In short, providers can help ensure that their teams meet requirements for proper care of LGBT residents by incorporating training and the other suggestions in this book into their daily operations. LGBT cultural competency can be cultivated in much the same way staff are trained to respect the religious, cultural, dietary, and linguistic preferences of residents from diverse backgrounds. For more information see Steelman 2018.

A 1986 study by the Institutes of Medicine found that many residents of nursing homes were being abused or receiving substandard care. This report lead to the passage of the Nursing Home Reform Act, part of the Omnibus Budget Reconciliation Act of 1987. This act requires that skilled nursing facilities who receive Medicare and Medicaid dollars must comply with the regulations of the act, and it also protects nursing home residents, regardless of sexual orientation or gender identity (42 U.S.C. § 1396r(a) and 42 U.S.C. § 1396r (b)(2); www.canhr.org/lgbt/relevant-laws.html).

The law also enumerates rights important to LGBT people. They include

- The right to freedom from abuse, mistreatment, and neglect;
- The right to freedom from physical restraints;
- The right to privacy;
- The right to accommodation of medical, physical, psychological, and social needs;
- The right to participate in resident and family groups;
- The right to be treated with dignity;
- The right to exercise self-determination;
- The right to communicate freely;
- The right to participate in the review of one's care plan and to be fully informed in advance about any changes in care, treatment, or change of status in the facility; and
- The right to voice grievances without discrimination or reprisal.

For example, the right to be free from abuse means that staff cannot harass or deny service to a resident because they are LGBT, the right to exercise self-determination gives residents the right to instruct staff on how they want to be dressed and addressed, and the right to privacy includes personal information like LGBT identity or HIV/AIDS status (National Long Term Care Ombudsman Resource Center 2018). LGBT older adults and advocates can apply the language of the Nursing Home Reform Act to their specific circumstances to argue for proper treatment, even if the language of the act does not explicitly outline sexual orientation and gender identity and expression as protected categories.

Finally, some professional licensing organizations, as well as state licensing requirements, are beginning to require training in LGBT cultural competency. You should check with your state and national licensing and professional associations for more information.

HEALTHCARE AND PRIVACY

The Patient Protection Affordable Care Act (often referred to as the Affordable Care Act or Obamacare) has a number of provisions that are particularly important for LGBT older adults. First, the ban on denying coverage or increasing premiums for pre-existing conditions is important for many people living with HIV/AIDS, as well as transgender older adults who are medically transitioning. Antiretroviral medications and hormone therapies can be expensive, and it is important that people making use of these medications have seamless access to them.

Section 1557 of the law prohibits discrimination on the basis of race, color, national origin, sex, age, or disability in "any health program or activity any part of which received funding from HHS; any health program or activity that HHS itself administers; and Health Insurance Marketplaces and all plans offered by issuers that participate in those Marketplaces" (OCR 2010).

This provision covers many senior living environments, including any provider who receives funding from Medicare or Medicaid, as well as hospitals and many skilled nursing and rehabilitation facilities. The Obama administration issued guidance stating that Section 1557's prohibition of discrimination on the basis of sex also protected people from discrimination on the basis of gender identity and sex stereotyping. The Trump administration has publicly stated that it plans to roll back that guidance.

The Health Information Portability and Accountability Act (HIPAA) is intended to protect a person's sensitive medical information. HIPAA protects information that could be relevant to a person's LGBT identity in at least two ways. First, if someone has HIV or AIDS that information is protected medical information. Again, not everyone with HIV/AIDS is LGBT, but because many people living with HIV/AIDS are also members of the LGBT community, disclosing a person's HIV/AIDS status without their consent may also out them as a member of the LGBT community. For more information on residents living with HIV/AIDS see Chapter 11.

Second, anything related to a person's medical transition is protected medical information, including surgical procedures or hormone therapy. Discussions about a resident's transition, or anything else about their bodily morphology, should be guided by HIPAA rules. Staff may not realize that information about a resident's transition is sensitive medical information, so proper training on when this information can be shared is an important way to ensure the privacy of your transgender residents.

CONTEMPORARY CONCERNS

In addition to some of the challenges described in the previous sections, in the United States it is the case that if a healthcare provider has a deeply held conviction that a healthcare procedure is not in line with their religious beliefs, they cannot be forced to participate in that procedure. There is a new push to expand Religious Freedom Restoration Act-style legislation, and many LGBT activists are concerned that policies intended to protect religious rights may be used to deny services to LGBT people. For more information on the intersection between LGBT older adults, aging services, and religious exemptions see the report *Dignity Denied: Religious Exemptions and LGBT Elder Services* at sageusa.org.

This information is constantly changing, so be sure to consult with advocacy organizations and legal experts to know the most up-to-date and accurate information about policy, laws, and regulations.

SUGGESTIONS

- Be aware of the laws, regulations, and protections that apply to your community or profession and how to comply with those laws and regulations.
- Information about a resident's LGBT identity should only be shared with their permission, or with a supervisor if that information impacts their care, health, or safety.
- Equip staff with information and resources about what to do if they feel a resident is experiencing discrimination.

FURTHER READING AND VIEWING

"Collecting Sexual Orientation and Gender Identity Data in Electronic Health Records" (www.lgbthealtheducation.org).

"Dignity Denied: Religious Exemptions and LGBT Elder Services" (www.sageusa.org/).

"Residents' Rights and the LGBT Community: Know YOUR Rights as a Nursing Home Resident" (http://ltcombudsman.org/uploads/files/support/lgbt-residents-rights-fact-sheet.pdf).

REFERENCES

CMS. 2017. "State Operations Manual: Appendix PP—Guidance to Surveyors for Long Term Care Facilities." Centers for Medicare and Medicaid Services. www.cms.gov/Regulations-and-Guidance/Guidance/Manuals/downloads/som107ap_pp_guidelines_ltcf.pdf.

HUD. n.d. "HUD LGBTQ Resources." *U.S. Department of Housing and Urban Development (HUD)*. Accessed November 22, 2018. www.hud.gov/LGBT_resources.

National Long Term Care Ombudsman Resource Center. 2018. "Residents' Rights and The LGBT Community: Know YOUR Rights as a Nursing Home Resident Updated 2018." The National Resource Center on LGBT Aging. http://ltcombudsman.org/uploads/files/support/lgbt-residents-rights-fact-sheet.pdf.

OCR. 2010. "Section 1557 of the Patient Protection and Affordable Care Act." *HHS.gov*. July 22, 2010. www.hhs.gov/civil-rights/for-individuals/section-1557/index.html.

Steelman, Rabbi Erica. 2018. "Person-Centered Care for LGBT Older Adults." *Journal of Gerontological Nursing* 44 (2): 3–5. https://doi.org/10.3928/00989134-20180110-01.

STRATEGIC PLANNING AND DIVERSIFYING THE BOARD

14

SUMMARY

What can your community do to make sure that your commitment to LGBT residents does not rely on specific staff or residents, but is integrated throughout the organization? This chapter examines different approaches to bringing your commitment to inclusion into your strategic and long-term planning processes and diversifying your organization's board to include LGBT perspectives.

OBJECTIVES

■ Identify ways to attract LGBT board members and educate your board on the importance of LGBT inclusion.
■ Set realistic and measurable goals that can guide your strategic plan.
■ Create mechanisms to solicit ongoing feedback.
■ Consider incorporating diversity and inclusion goals into employee coaching and performance evaluations.

SPARKING PASSION ACROSS THE STAFF

When I cold-call a senior center or senior living community it can be difficult to explain why LGBT inclusion is important because many providers do not think they work with LGBT older people. I can cite statistics or try to explain why their residents may be closeted, but if they are not receptive it is hard to get in the door. I, and many of my fellow advocates, therefore rely on invitations from passionate staff with the experience or vision to understand the importance of LGBT inclusion. Sometimes that person is the executive director; other times they are a nurse, programming assistant, or volunteer. These individuals are essential champions to lead efforts at becoming more inclusive and I could not do my work without them.

That said, having only one committed advocate within an organization puts any effort to address LGBT inclusion on shaky footing, no matter how invested the advocate is in the process. After all, what happens if that person gets a new job or retires? What if they have only limited influence or authority to make changes within the organization? Individual passion and charisma are essential components of starting the process of larger structural changes, but in the long term creating a positive environment for LGBT residents requires that commitment be woven into the fabric of the community.

EXPLAINING INCLUSION TO THE BOARD

The first step to addressing LGBT inclusion for many organizations is getting board members to understand the necessity of investing time, energy, and resources into these efforts. You and your team have the best sense of what your board will find compelling. The following are useful ways I have found for framing the issues and communicating them.

The moral case

Many of your board members have a personal connection to aging services, person-directed care, and providing for the needs of older adults and other vulnerable populations. Most people, when they first hear about the challenges facing LGBT elders, immediately react by saying "Wow, I've never thought about that!" If you can educate the board on the hidden and pressing needs of LGBT residents, that can create a compelling moral and emotional motivation to think seriously about making the structural changes outlined in this text and to support staff in creating an inclusive space. Consider showing the trailer for the film *Gen Silent* or reading some of the case studies and testimonials in the report "LGBT Older Adults in Long-Term Care Facilities: Stories from the Field." These are impactful messaging tools to communicate the urgency and importance of committing to LGBT inclusion.

The family case

If board members are doubtful that they have, or will have, LGBT residents, it is helpful to point out that many current and future residents have LGBT family members. My parents are not LGBT, but they would never live in a place where I did not feel comfortable bringing my male partner with me to visit them. We do not want our communities to be islands or retreats separated from the geographic and cultural communities that surround them, and as our society gets increasingly diverse and supportive of LGBT identities it is important that senior living does the same.

The staff case

This training is information that staff need to do their jobs well. Not many staffers in aging services have been trained on LGBT inclusion, so it is a way to invest in your staff, increase their skills, and let them know they are working for an innovative company that supports their professional development. Members of your staff may be LGBT or have LGBT family members, and the community's commitment to being inclusive will go a long way toward making those staffers feel included and even proud to be a part of the company.

BOX 14.1   REBECCA HILL'S STORY

When I interviewed here I was narrowing my job search between the Carlotta and another employer. My interview included a lot of information about the property and the interviewer did mention the SAGECare LGBT training program. I have to say the SAGE program is definitely a wonderful program. I think most people, including myself, don't really give much thought to retirement life, maybe because it seems so far away for us. As a lesbian woman who has been with my wife for 28 years, the SAGE program has given me a good feeling and I know that we can find a retirement community that welcomes everyone. It makes me very proud to tell people my employer is a part of the SAGE program.

Rebecca Hill, Executive Chef
The Fountains at the Carlotta
Palm Desert, California

The financial case

If all else fails, there is, of course, a financial case to be made. Demonstrating a commitment to LGBT elders is a new and innovative idea in the industry, and can be a way for your community to distinguish itself from competitors. As noted elsewhere, many LGBT people are economically vulnerable, but there are also wealthy members of the LGBT community who have considerable purchasing power. Attracting that market can increase occupancy, reaching potential residents who otherwise might not have considered your community.

Given that many LGBT people are closeted and most communities do not track LGBT identity in their census documents it can be difficult to determine the return on investment from becoming more inclusive. To that end, inclusive intake as discussed in Chapter 3 can be an important way to measure and report back to the board on the impact of these changes. I suggest you create a consistent way to record if your efforts at LGBT inclusion are having a positive impact on occupancy. This might include interviews with new residents about why they chose your community, a survey of what people find most appealing at the community, or training staff to make note when residents discuss LGBT inclusion in a positive way.

ATTRACTING LGBT BOARD MEMBERS

LGBT communities are just as diverse as our society at large, and no single LGBT person can speak for the experiences and perspectives of all LGBT people. That said, bringing openly LGBT-identified people onto your board and into your staff can help ensure that LGBT perspectives are voiced at all levels of the organization.

Of course, no one should be installed on your organization's board simply because they are LGBT. Rather, when considering potential new board members, the perspectives LGBT candidates can bring to organization governance should be thought of as one particular—and particularly important—qualification that recommends them, in addition to all of their other skills, credentials, and experience. The question to ask yourself is: how can we ensure that LGBT people are represented in the pool of potential board members from which we will select the most qualified applicants?

In addition to leveraging your current board's personal and professional networks, consider building relationships with the following types of groups:

- LGBT community centers;
- LGBT equality groups;
- LGBT chambers of commerce;
- HIV/AIDS advocacy organizations or providers;
- LGBT-affirming mental health clinics;
- University or campus LGBT centers.

Reaching out to these groups will increase the likelihood of finding LGBT people who may make good additions to your board. It is also important to note that due to discrimination and years of unequal taxation, many LGBT people—especially LGBT people of color and transgender people—have, on average, lower incomes and less wealth than white and cisgender people. If board members are expected to donate and fundraise this may be a barrier for candidates. Consider relaxing those requirements or adding additional board members who are expected to provide strategic vision and ideas but are not pressured to donate or fundraise.

STRATEGIC PLANNING

One place where a diverse board and community staff can begin to have a strong impact on your organization is the strategic planning process. While it is beyond the scope of this chapter to discuss the broader theories of strategic planning, there are a number of ways to incorporate LGBT inclusion into whatever process your community undertakes.

As you begin to craft your narratives, goals, and strategies, think of places where you can include specific wording that highlights LGBT residents. For example, consider the following goal and two strategies for achieving it. The goal does not specifically mention LGBT people, but both strategies contain language that makes it clear the goal applies to them:

> Goal: Become a place where residents, their family members, loved ones, and members of the wider community want to spend time.
> Strategy 1: Ensure that our visitation policies and public-facing messaging clearly communicate that our conception of "family" is not limited to biological or legal family members, but also includes friends and other chosen family.
> Strategy 2: Start a speaker and film series addressing current national conversations around such issues as civil rights and the Black Lives Matter movement, faith and religion, LGBT pride and inclusion, climate change and ecological conservation, or other topics of interest to residents and community members.

The first strategy is explicitly intended to address the unique family structures and networks that support many LGBT older adults. The second strategy focuses on bringing people from the broader community in to interact with residents, and the addition of LGBT-specific topics can help normalize them by demonstrating that events like those are supported by staff members and the organization's board.

For more examples of how the strategic planning process can be made more LGBT-inclusive see the guide "Strengthen Your State and Local Aging Plan: A Practical Guide for Expanding the Inclusion of LGBT Older Adults," available at www.lgbtagingcenter.org

SEEING SUCCESSES AND NEXT CHALLENGES

A strategic plan is both a map for the next several years and a set of outcomes or benchmarks against which to measure progress along the way. Most people are familiar with creating SMART goals (Specific, Measurable, Achievable, Relevant, Time-Bound) but what about goals that are specific to creating a more welcoming environment for LGBT residents? Do not be shy about making very specific goals—they will help you determine whether your plan is being successfully executed.

BOX 14.2 LGBT-SPECIFIC STRATEGIC GOALS

Creating these goals may involve taking the best practices found throughout this book and applying specific measurements or timelines.

Goals measured by timeline or deadline

Implement LGBT cultural competency training in this fiscal year.
Create one LGBT-specific program or event each quarter.

Goals measured by specific numbers

Increase the percentage of residents who openly identify as LGBT.
Increase the number of board members who openly identify as LGBT.
Form a partnership with one new LGBT advocacy or community organization.

Goals measured by qualitative feedback

Enhance the public perception of our community as LGBT-inclusive, as evaluated by focus groups and surveys.
Create and implement a "community climate and culture" survey for residents and staff. Deliver the survey annually and measure any changes.

Board meetings, staff meetings, newsletters, and town halls are all excellent opportunities for gauging progress toward these goals. They are moments to both celebrate successes and identify obstacles or challenges.

Diversifying both your staff and your organization's board and setting concrete and specific goals around LGBT inclusion will help ensure that the work described in this book does not fall entirely on you or a few other particularly motivated members of your organization. Instead, it will become a part of the fabric of your community.

SUGGESTIONS

- Work to recruit qualified board members who are also LGBT or have strong connections to LGBT communities.
- Set measurable, time-bound goals to track your progress, creating a more inclusive community and attracting LGBT residents.
- Build partnerships with local LGBT organizations and advocacy groups.

FURTHER READING AND VIEWING

Gen Silent (film) (www.theclowdergroup.com/gensilent).
"LGBT Older Adults in Long-Term Care Facilities: Stories from the Field" (www.justiceinaging.org/lgbt-older-adults-in-long-term-care-facilities-stories-from-the-field-2/).
"Strengthen Your State and Local Aging Plan: A Practical Guide for Expanding the Inclusion of LGBT Older Adults" (www.lgbtagingcenter.org/resources/resource.cfm?r=865).

CONCLUSION

It starts with you!

LGBT aging activists are a committed and fierce group, and we could not do the work we do without equally passionate allies and supporters. I hope this book has given you actionable strategies for incorporating LGBT inclusion into your everyday work, as well as ideas for how to introduce structural changes that will make your community more welcoming to LGBT older adults.

Much of what I have discussed in this book centers around expanding our perspectives so that we can avoid making assumptions about our residents. Active listening, open-ended questions, and repeating back the words and phrases that you hear residents using are essential components of creating a more welcoming environment.

This is particularly important because many LGBT older people are afraid to be open and may be hiding their identities until they see clear signals that they will be treated with respect. Having LGBT-inclusive visitation policies, nondiscrimination statements, and a set of community standards that expressly mention LGBT inclusion all send a positive message to current and future residents. These policies, when coupled with staff training and LGBT programming, can show that your community respects and welcomes LGBT people and their family members.

None of us is perfect, and there will be challenges along the way. Every one of us will make mistakes, say the wrong thing, make a situation awkward, or need to navigate hurt and conflict. These conversations may feel stressful or uncomfortable. But as I have said, it is impossible to know who will push back and who will emerge as your champions until you have started these discussions in your community. The conversation starts with you, and it isn't until we all begin discussing LGBT inclusion that we will see the road ahead.

Remember too that this work is fun, interesting, and urgently important. Senior living staff have the opportunity to help create places where everyone can feel at home, and even the smallest changes can have positive ripple-effects that we might not ever fully understand or appreciate. You and your team might make all of the changes I have suggested in this book, implement every best practice, and still never have a resident come out. That's OK. Trust that people are noticing, and that even if they do not come out publicly, you are having a positive impact on their lives.

Be bold, be brave, and let the strength, resiliency, and humor of our LGBT elders inspire you in this work. This is not zero-sum—becoming a more inclusive space for LGBT elders will create a more positive environment for all residents, staff members, families, and friends.

INDEX

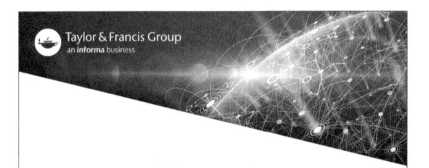

Printed in the United States
by Baker & Taylor Publisher Services